CW01513110

The Com_
Guide to Bunion
Problems

Is surgery always necessary?

David R Tollafield

With

Tim E Kilmartin

Images used within this book, except those cited, have been licensed through Shutterstock.com

Cover by Petya Tsankova

Published by Busypencilcase Communications. Est. 2015

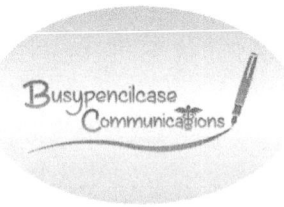

Foreword

To borrow a popular advertising slogan, this book does exactly what it says on the tin. I was fortunate enough to read the first version (*Bunion, Hallux Valgus Behind the Scenes*) released in 2019. If I had to sum up this second updated and extended version in one word, I'd say '*comprehensive*'.

This new edition is, without doubt, an extensive tour de force of all thing's bunion.

David Tollafield teamed up with Dr Tim Kilmartin bringing together two experts with 60 years' experience of caring for patients and fixing bunions.

It's fair to say few, if any, will have contributed more to the development of podiatric surgery and bunion correction in the UK. And what a result; this book leaves no stone unturned in helping patients understand what a bunion is, how to manage the condition themselves before delving into the surgical options, surgical risks and complications.

Expertise is all well and good, but the authors have chosen to include multiple testimonials from people who have been through bunion surgery. We can all, patients and clinicians alike, learn a great deal from listening to the lived experience of those who have already been through treatment.

Although this book is explicitly written for patients, I would commend it to a wider audience including podiatrists, nurses, trainees, podiatric surgeons and orthopaedic surgeons.

Anthony Maher, FRCPodS

Preface

THE COMPLETE PATIENT GUIDE TO BUNION
PROBLEMS. *IS SURGERY ALWAYS NECESSARY?*

We are excited to create a new guide for patients and
healthcare professionals that spotlights this common
condition. The first version, *Bunion Hallux Valgus: Behind
the Scenes*, was published in 2019. Although the title of this
book has changed, this second edition has been updated and
packed with more images. It is supported by an extensive
section on patient feedback (Part IV) that is unlikely to be
found elsewhere, along with clinical explanations. Where
possible, we have tried to justify each comment with
reputable scientific evidence. Footnotes provide further
explanation and contain links to sites of value. Any images
containing product references are not featured to advertise
promote or recommend, but should be taken to exemplify a
particular design or modality.

This guide is considered 'complete' not because it has
everything ever written about bunions but because we have
offered two smaller e-books — *Understanding & Managing
Your Bunion*, and *What You Need to Know about Bunion
Surgery – patient stories of actual events[1]*. If you have
bought this book you will already have both.

Dr Tim Kilmartin brings additional expertise and practical
advice on surgery. We have over sixty years of clinical
experience between us, and one of our principal roles was
managing bunion (hallux valgus) problems. Who better to
write a book, especially when one author has undergone foot
surgery?

---

[1] These two eBooks will be available from March 2025.

The Complete Patient Guide To Bunion Problems.

With well over a hundred operations described for bunion problems, numerous books, and published articles on the internet, it makes sense to place information in one place. As podiatrists, we have seen the value of quality advice in helping people make decisions that suit their needs and helping them on their journey, removing false expectations and inspiring patients with this condition to make the right decisions about their treatment.

We believe no one should be denied access to information, which often means reflecting on the downsides as well as the positive sides of care. Using patient diaries and worldwide queries from the UK and USA, this edition broadens many common questions, sometimes before surgery, sometimes after.

Patients should only decide which approach to take after understanding the facts and discussing this with their foot surgeon. In addition to footnotes, the book's format includes an index, valuable links to videos, and interactive patient comments.

We hope that our book will appeal to everyone, whether you live in the UK, the USA, or another part of the world.

David R Tollafield FRCPodS, MSc, BSc, DPodM, FRCPodM
& Tim Kilmartin PhD, FRCPodS

January 2025

Tollafield DR & Kilmartin TE

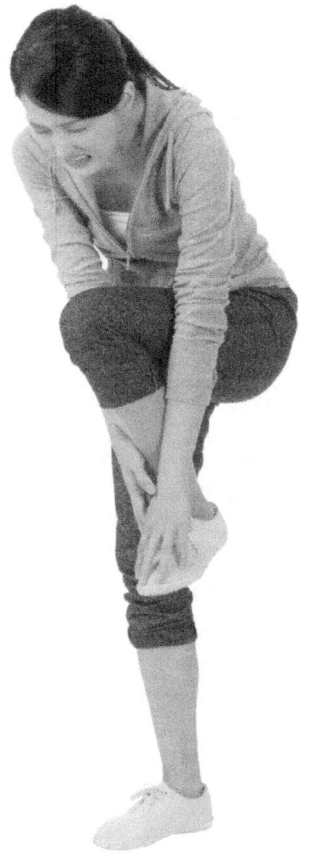

The bunion is not just a condition affecting the aged patient.

My family doctor says he doesn't know the answers to my questions, and I don't want to make another mistake or have fusion if my feet can be fixed. I really value your opinion, and I have not been so fortunate to find someone here like you that puts out so much helpful information for everyone and answers questions and comments at the end of articles.
Gail —a desperate patient.

Although I'm used to approaching everything from a textbook point of view, the patient's perspective revealed that there's much more to decision-making than just focusing solely on the clinical and anatomical causes for action. It wasn't structured like a textbook but provided the same depth of knowledge, but it was much more enjoyable to read and easier to understand.
Sahiba Atwal—Final Year Podiatry Student, University of Southampton.

Contents

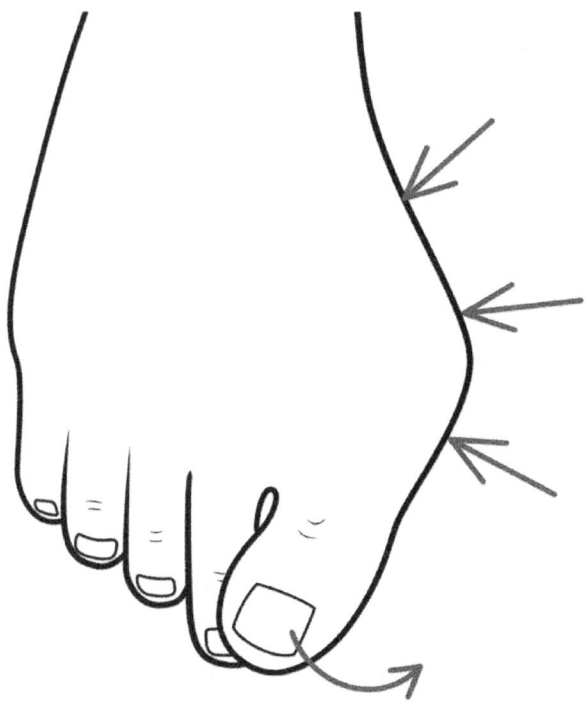

The bunion may appear a simple concern but the problem is both complex in terms of mechanics and its progressive nature. The first toe, (hallux) widens the foot and adds to footwear fitting difficulties. Pressure causes skin damage but the story does not ends there and needs a book to complete the story...

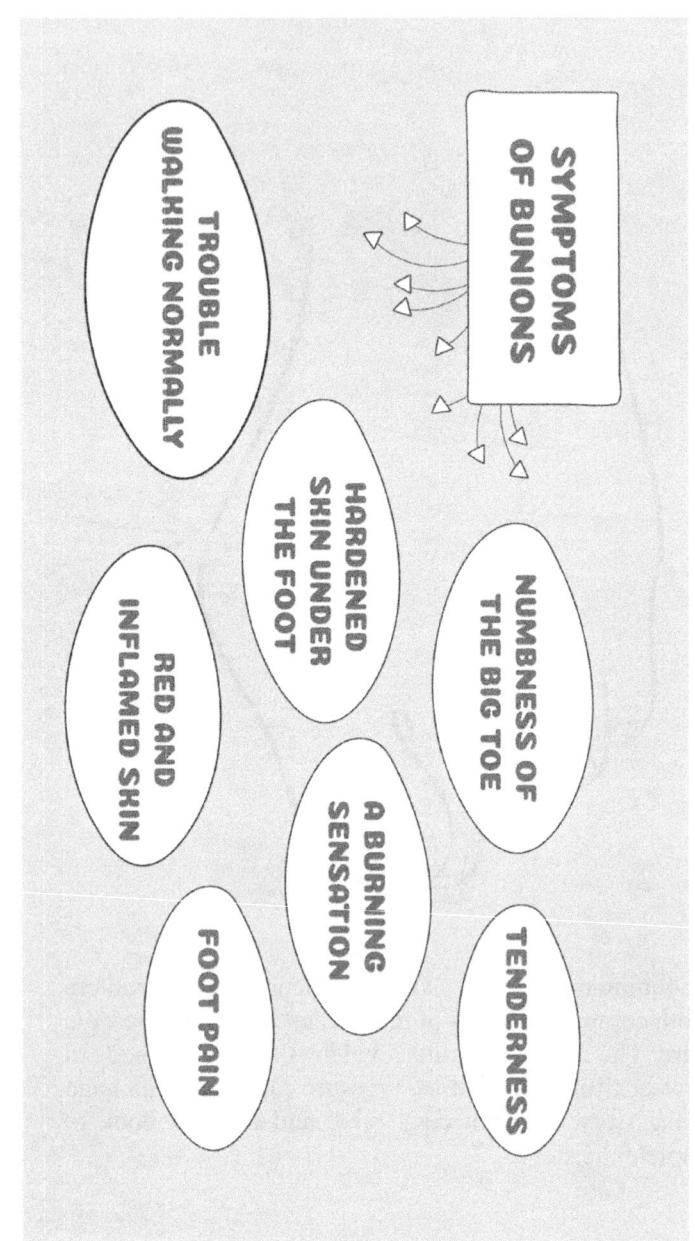

Introduction

So, why buy this book?

How do you select the best fruit? Someone has to tell you first which fruit is best suited for eating, or your other choice is to taste it and hope for the best. Oscar Wilde suggested,

> *If you learn from your own experience*
> *you are clever, if you learn from*
> *someone else's you are a genius.*

Our book is intended to inform and support the reader with reliable, qualified advice from experienced people you can trust at a pocket-sized price. As with all guide books, the title means just that—a guide to offer advice but does not necessarily fit every situation.

Books on the bunion often make false promises, and advice sheets can provide a sterile view of the realities. Some of the material has been taken from the website consultingfootpain.co.uk, which patients have interacted with since its inception over ten years ago. This provides a valuable manual of personal viewpoints with questions and answers.

Some books suggest exercise will cure the deformity, devices to change the toe position, and foot inserts sold to suggest the deformity can be prevented. We need to distil some of these myths and separate misleading information. One of the complaints seen from reader feedback on Amazon is the promotion of a book to drive patients to the author's clinic. Our book is impartial in all respects, advocating orthopaedic specialists as well as podiatrists qualified to perform surgery.

Where possible, we have responded to patient queries from our clinical experience and do not suggest surgery as the only solution to the problem. Hence, there are many explanations regarding fitting and stretching shoes, skincare, and generally living with the deformity in harmony.

Writing about a common complaint like a bunion seems pointless without providing a balanced view. There needs to be more clarity about whether to have something done. If you are still contemplating bunion surgery, please read this book first. If you want to consider self-help, we will cover this important subject. If surgery is not for you, we will discuss the alternatives.

Terminology has been minimised, except for terms that may be encountered along the way.

Part I: Defines the problem and covers all the causes referring to basic anatomy. You will understand the nuances of the condition hallux valgus (bunion).

Part II: Dedicated to self-help and non-surgical intervention

Part III: Surgery, decision-making, consent, complications, admission and recovery.

Part IV: Patient-focused material includes diaries and common questions. It focuses on behind-the-scenes and problem-solving and offers recovery tips.

Case histories and clinical comments are provided in designated boxes.

Confusing tips need sifting:

- *'Go to him or her, don't go to him or her.'*
- *'I was made worse!'*
- *'It took so long to recover.'*
- *'I was back on my feet after 10 days.'*
- *'You don't need surgery.'*
- *'Try this splint or that method.'*

Helpful or not, patients are guided by what they know and influenced by who they trust. If you've bought this book, we will take you to a level beyond the advice your GP can give and fill in some gaps.

When it comes to treatment, it is reasonable that surgery should be the last option. Education and effective communication covering the pros and cons of surgery are nine-tenths of the battle. After this, the choice becomes easier, provided that information has realistic evidence to support any discussion. You cannot make an effective choice unless you have sufficient information.

These are the bits that people may not tell you; for example, after surgery, haemorrhoids (piles) may worsen, and you may experience side effects from pain medication and strained inter-partner relationships – just a few examples from our patient diaries.

Silverman, Kurtz and Draper[2], in their book Skills for Communicating with Patients (2013), tell us that only 53% of doctors provide such information despite a clear desire for information amongst patients. Although we have no additional statistics, it is likely that since 2013, most NHS and independent clinicians will offer advice sheets, hopefully not photocopied, until the letters become bleached and illegible! Where factsheets are used, the parts essential to the treating clinician may differ significantly from the elements the patient wants or needs. Our belief lies behind the idea that there is a need for more detail than that gained from factsheets alone; be reassured, factsheets still have value.

The quality of information has never been more critical as legal imperatives have changed the scene, thrusting patients into the light of compensation. The standards of the day never remain stationary. While this book is written for patients, foot health clinicians and medical doctors who are at the forefront of referrals will also benefit from the content that supports any clinical discussion. Patients never more so than today need to achieve the most from their face-to-face time with healthcare providers. While we do not advocate surgery for every bunion and feel there are other options, management often falls to surgery. Inevitably, some bias exists in the second half of this book toward surgery.

---

[2] Silverman,J, Kurtz,S, Draper,J. Skills for Communicating with Patients. CRC Press. Third Edition. 2013

Part I

In this section, we will ensure that you understand the difference between a bunion and hallux valgus, the likely causes, the anatomy and mechanics as part of the role of the great toe, and the problems that arise with the development of an issue that affects other parts of the foot.

The foot influences the skeleton above, and so the deformity becomes more complex than just a single problem associated with a bony projection.

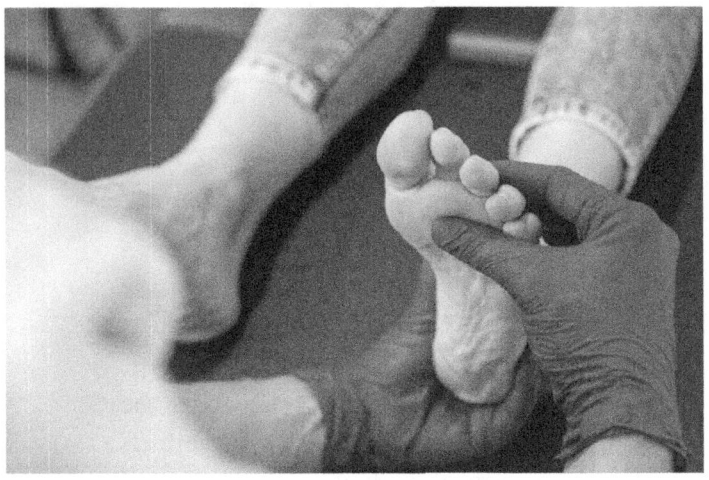

Diagnosing Hallux Valgus

Patients ask many questions and should be encouraged to do so. If you read this book or dip into its content before a consultation, your questions will be better supported by knowing what to ask, who to ask, and when to ask without fear of a hostile reaction. Clinicians are there to guide you, advise you and respect your decision. They do not, nor should they, pressurise you into any particular treatment.

Depression

It might seem unusual, but hallux valgus is not a condition that immediately assumes a relationship with depression.

López (2015)[3] published an interesting article in the journal 'Mental Health Nursing'. He used a questionnaire-scoring system called the Beck Depression Inventory (BDI). Taking one hundred and two participants, he found that 38% had depression associated with the BDI criteria.

Based on the definition of disease[4], hallux valgus contains the element of deformity and impairs normal function. The first part of this book will explain how foot function is impaired.

The Beck inventory included some of the criteria that as clinicians we see but may not relate to depression in hallux valgus—

- Loss of hope.
- Inability to enjoy life.
- Negative self-image.
- Unable to work.
- Disturbed sleep.

The list includes sixteen other questions. Scores under ten suggest no depression, and the highest score is sixty-three, pointing to severe depression. The study was also linked to age, gender and location. Photographs were used to determine the severity of the deformity.

Within the sample, females predominated at 70.6% compared to 29.4% of males. As the deformity increased, so did the BDI score. López, a professor at the University of

---

[3] López DL, Fernández JM, Iglesias ME, Castro CÁ, Lobo CC, Galván JR, de Bengoa Vallejo RB. Influence of depression in a sample of people with hallux valgus. Int J Ment Health Nurs. 2016 Dec;25(6):574-578. doi: 10.1111/inm.12196. Epub 2016 Feb 19. PMID: 26892262.
[4] A condition of the living animal or plant body or of one of its parts that impairs normal functioning and is typically manifested by distinguishing signs and symptoms. Webster Accessed September 2024.

Coruna in Spain, worked with podiatrists and physiotherapists. The authors highlight the importance of body image, especially among women with footwear impacting on image. They go on to state that—

> The loss of choice in footwear as a consequence of the disease impacted negatively on emotions and well-being and was found to reduce the self-perceived quality of life.

We need to start at the beginning and discuss what a bunion is or is not.

What Exactly is a Bunion?

A bunion is the enlarged shape associated with the big toe's main joint.

Defining the bunion as the main problem is slightly more complicated, and we must apply the Bunion Test. The **Bunion Test** helps identify the extent of the deformity shown in the right-hand picture. We note the deviation angle or hallux valgus angle.

By covering the bump with your hand, the toe position is shown to be within normal limits. The toe is only slightly angled, which is insufficient to define it as having a valgus position.

The left-hand illustration suggests this is a significant deformity when the distortion arises on the medial side, that is, the foot's inner side.

While the bunion is the bump, the deformity comprises the enlarged size and the shifting of the great toe into a windswept direction.

Valgus is the deviation that can be 5-15° and considered within normal limits. It would indeed not be regarded as appropriate for surgery alone. The first toe is called the 'hallux'.

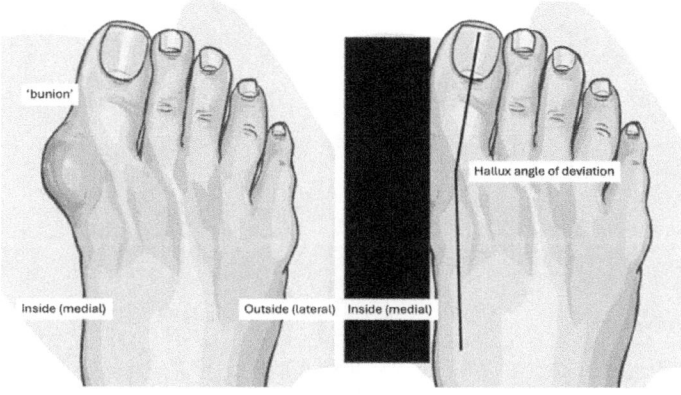

Fig.1.1. The Bunion Test to identify hallux valgus from a bunion. The enlarged side of the foot in the left picture. While the toe knocks the second toe, the deformity remains small under the standard 15°.

When is a Bunion Called Hallux Valgus (HV)?

Hallux valgus, or HV, is where the first toe is displaced. The bump may still exist, but the buckling toe being windswept to the foot's outer side (lateral) complicates the problem. Pressure is placed against the second toe Fig.1.2 left foot.

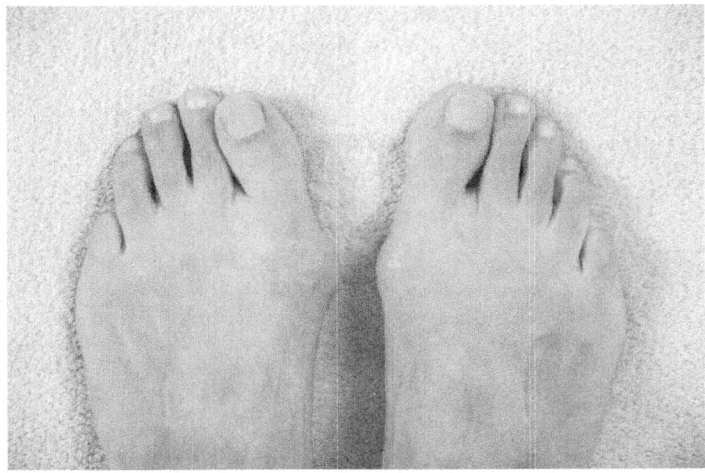

Fig.1.2. The left foot shows contact with the second toe (hallux valgus), with an accompanying bunion on the right foot. Sometimes the difference is subtle.

Once the great toe—known as the hallux—knocks the second toe, four changes can arise over a period of time. The hallux:—

- Rotates, as shown in Fig.1.4.
- Overrides the second toe. (As in Fig.1.2 above).
- Dislocates the second toe off course—Fig. 1.5.
- Underrides the second toe and may push it off course—Fig. 1.5.

Traditionally, clinicians consider a hallux valgus present when the measured deformity lies above 20°. We will learn that even higher positions of displacement create few problems for many people who live without requiring any intervention.

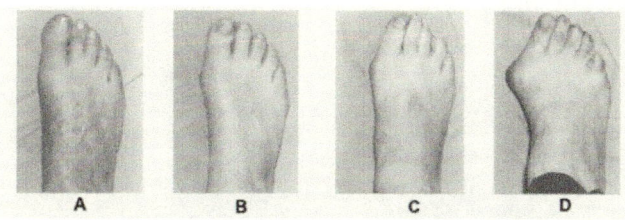

Fig.1.3. Progressive Hallux Valgus deformity over time. Normal (A) to severe (D), where the foot broadens.

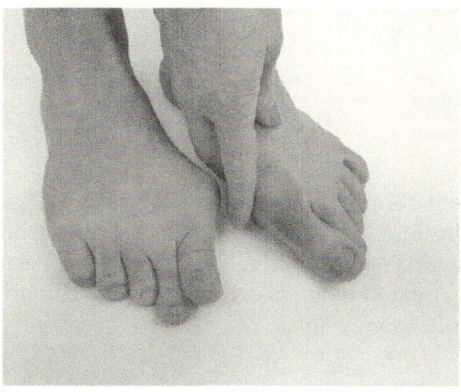

Fig.1.4. Two deformities in one. Rotation of the big toe.

The patient's finger lies over the distended joint of the bunion, Fig.1.4, but both feet show rotation of the hallux. The giveaway sign is that the toenail no longer faces upward but rests at an angle. Patients frequently feel discomfort from the groove where the nail squashes against the shoe when such a deformity exists.

A bunion may present as a soft spongy joint, where a sac called a cyst may arise. In other cases, the hardness is formed from the enlarged bone, called an exostosis. When the joint is displaced, it implies the two bones are no longer aligned, and the hallux has slipped sideways. To illustrate misalignment, let's look at the following figure where the hallux deformity is severe.

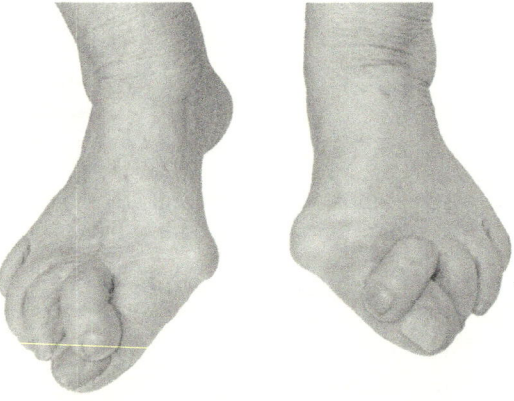

Fig.1.5. Severe deformity in both feet. The hallux has swept over and now hits the third toe. The second toe has been pushed up and is no longer aligned with the joint. The left hallux is rotated more than the right. A hard bunion is seen and mainly comprises bone rather than a soft, spongy bursa.

Subluxation & Dislocation

When the joint becomes misaligned, the two bones making the joint fail to sit correctly and are considered to form a partial dislocation, also known as subluxation. Some toes can increase their position to 90 degrees and push all the smaller toes out of the way (Fig.1.6—severe). By doing nothing as we age, patients find they are in trouble because all the toes start dislocating creating pressure against the shoe.

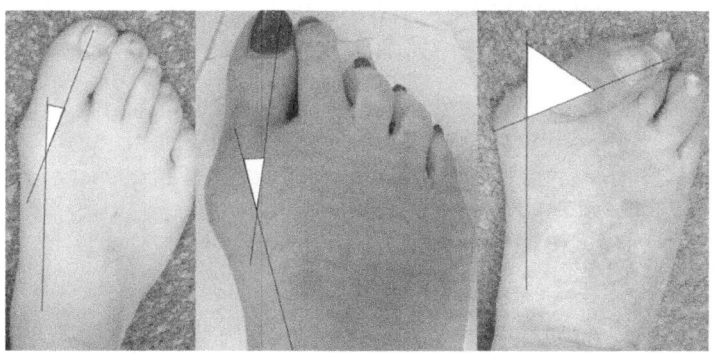

Fig.1.6. Three examples of subluxation with increasing deformity angles - from left to right—mild, moderate and severe. (Tollafield 2019). The angle marked is the hallux valgus angle.

For the sake of simplicity, all references in this guidebook will use mild and moderate, with severe in the context of multiple complications with more than one toe. At this stage, the patient may ask, "Should I need my other toes managed?" In addition to the deformity, skin damage arises, which will be dealt with separately. As the skin stretches, it is exposed to shoe pressure. Again, a question might arise—"I don't have trouble with my bunion or hallux, but the skin is painful."

Joint Pain

When considering the condition of a bunion or hallux valgus in isolation, the inside of the joint, the synovial cellular membrane may form a reactive inflammation within the joint's lining.

The bone enlarges for two reasons.

- The bone itself is irritated and lays down more bone cells.
- The bracing ligaments stretch inside the joint and pull against the bone, causing liquid-filled craters (bone cysts).

The sac described and shown in Fig 1.7. may arise from inside the joint and within the deeper layers of the cyst, which may be due to a ganglion or bursa. These cysts Fig 8—look similar from the outside but appear differently under a microscope.

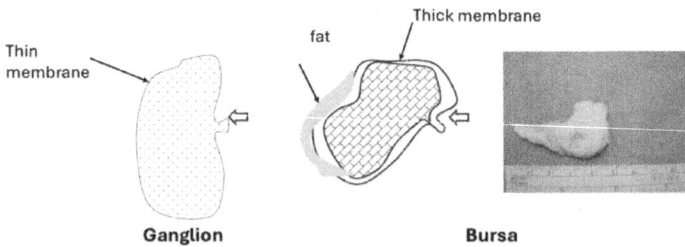

Fig.1.7. provides a schematic illustration of the two soft cysts and an inset image of a bursa removed from under the first metatarsal. (Tollafield 2024)

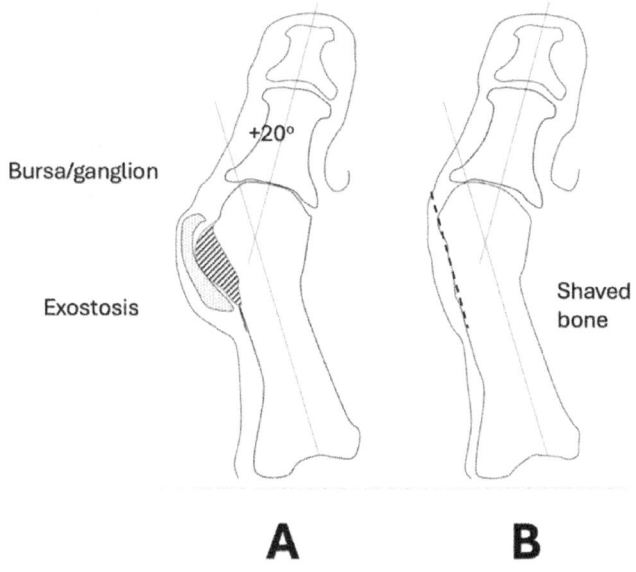

Fig.1.8. Shows two sets of bones and joints. A – soft swelling and B – surgery removes the cyst and exostosis (shaded).

While the deformity is mild, the bone has adapted (shaded), forming new bone cells that build up the bunion's size as an exostosis. In A, the soft tissue bursa/ganglion overlies the exostosis. The exostosis is the bump formed from excessive bone cells called osteocytes. An excess of bone, especially around joints, is termed osteophytes.

In B, the exostosis has been shaved, alleviating some skin pressure but not correcting the underlying deformity. There are several self-help methods to protect the skin and pressure from shoes.

When discussing bunions, we now know we must be clear about whether the toe experiences pain because of inflammation, soft tissue buildup from a bursa/ganglion, or whether an exostosis is causing pressure.

If the lesser toes are dislocated or subluxed, shoe fit may pose a problem. As the hallux deviates, it may give rise to more than one problem, which is determined as mild, moderate and severe hallux valgus.

Older patients with thin and fragile skin and poor circulation are at greater risk from skin damage and healing concerns.

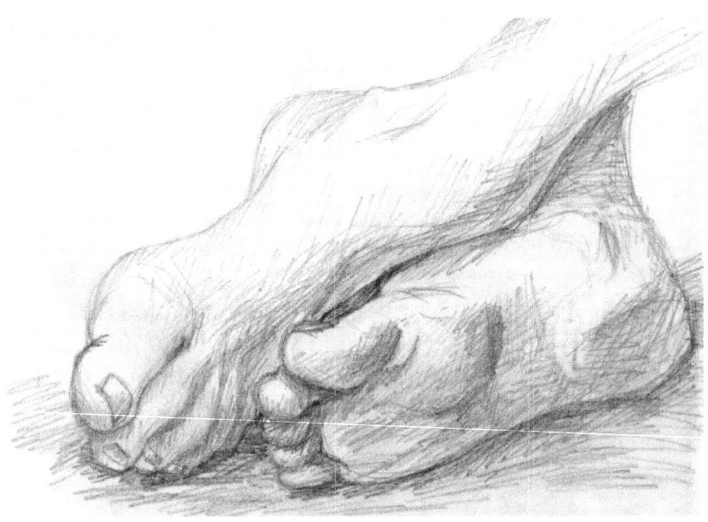

Anatomy & Altering Foot Mechanics

Understanding the anatomy and what is going wrong (pathology) is helpful. Consider this a map toward better understanding your condition.

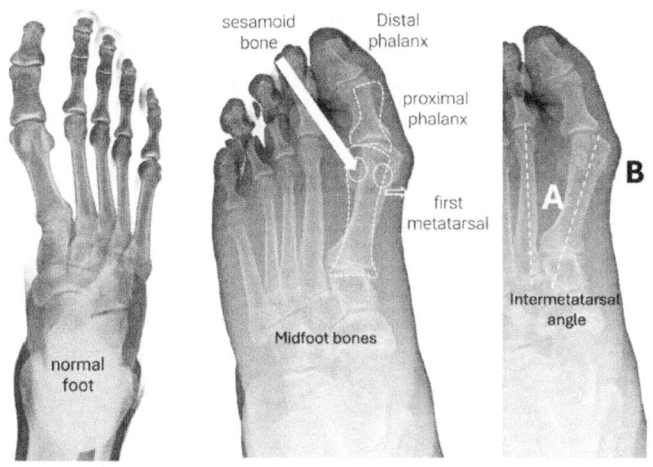

Fig.1.9. Anatomy of a Hallux deformity as shown by X-ray.

Anatomy refers to the parts of the foot, namely the bones. The mechanics is how the anatomy functions smoothly in association with the remaining skeleton. This is only a small part of the story when describing the first toe joint.

No one expects the lay reader to expand upon that understanding, although you can read several books that will improve your knowledge.[5] Fig.1.9 shows us how we might assess the foot using an X-ray when presented with the problem. An X-ray allows us to view the alignment, bone length and its relationship with other bones. You will see the sesamoid bones marked as circles. These tiny structures provide an essential effect on the stability of the toe.

Clinicians talk about pathology, which implies abnormal changes in the body usually caused by disease. An imbalance of the mechanics can still lead to pathology as localised injury. In Fig. 1.9, angle A is the intermetatarsal angle, which should be small. Once the angle increases, point B forms a bump, and our bunion appears as a projection. The higher the angle between the first metatarsal and its neighbour, the more the toe is pushed over.

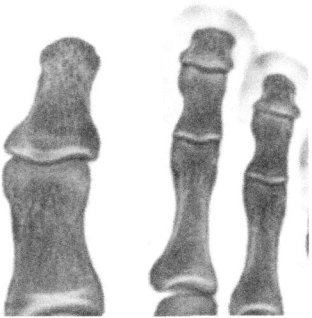

Fig. 1.10. Phalanges are toe bones. The left is called the hallux.

As foot surgeons, we grade how much the big toe drifts. However, mild, moderate, and severe conditions simplify our discussion. The first toe joint is called the metatarsophalangeal joint (MTPJ), which comprises two bones, the metatarsal and phalanx, separated by a cartilage-covered cap on each bone. The cartilage allows smooth gliding movement. Most mtpj's move upwards by 60-70°,

---

[5] An Introduction to the Adult Foot & Its Common Problems in the Adult. Tollafield D R 2023. Amazon Books.

providing good push-off movement, ensuring a regular walking pattern. The two phalanges— proximal and a distal bone. Together, they form the hallux. There is a joint between these smaller bones called the interphalangeal joint (IPJ). The first metatarsal is the thickest of all the five metatarsals in the forefoot. The ipj only has a downward movement of some 20-50°.

When we walk, our body weight transfers across the outside of the foot to the first toe. As the heel lifts, the big toe and the hallux, combined from these two bones, are held on the ground by strong (flexor) tendons. The powerful flexor tendon (Fig.1.11) works from the leg, around the ankle and inserts into the hallux. Two bones called sesamoids aid the tendon's mechanical efficiency, allowing the toe to remain stable as the heel lifts. In addition to the tendon, sesamoids, and bones, fat pads cushion the foot in two areas. The main body weight is distributed through these two locations. For the first toe to function correctly, the first mtpj should be aligned. The dotted outline of the metatarsal shows the correct position against the bones represented by the X-ray (Fig.1.9) of the foot.

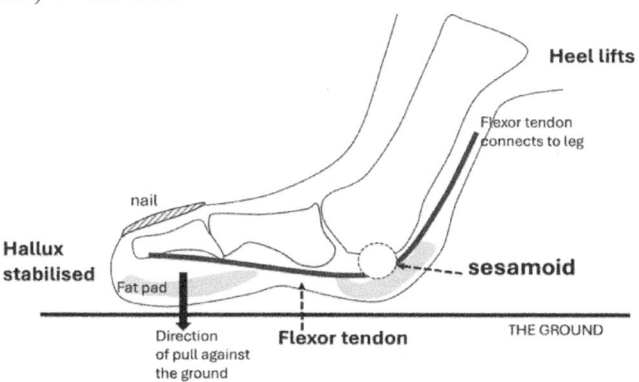

Fig.1.11. First mtpj working when the heel lifts during walking.

Muscle Influence on the First Toe

It is essential to understand why some treatments fail and some succeed. More will be covered under self-care and non-surgical treatment.

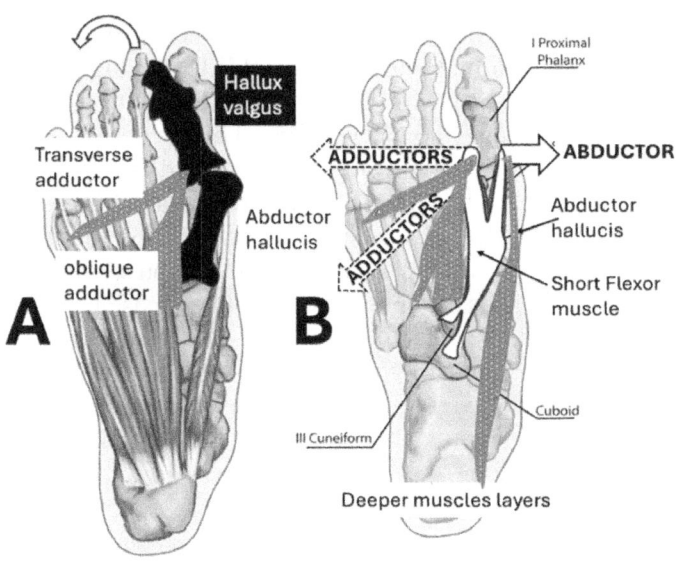

Fig. 1.12. A – the two adductor muscles are shown, pulling the great toe over. B – the short flexor muscle loses its function if the toe starts to subluxate, as in A.

Consider your position on the edge of a swimming pool at a point where you lean forward. You fall into the water once your body has reached a point of no return.

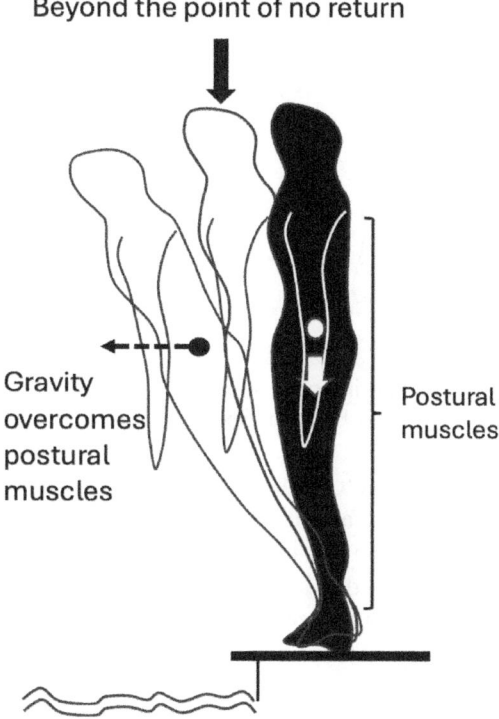

Fig.1.13. Swimming Pool analogy: gravity over muscle power as the centre of mass shifts forward.

In much the same way, if the toe reaches a point where there is less contact between the bones, the outer muscle can overpower the toe joint stability. Severe hallux valgus deformities are beyond help from conservative care.

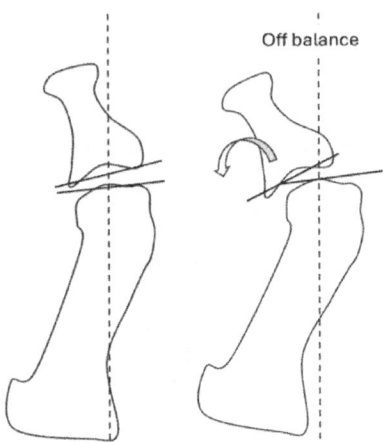

Off balance

Fig.1.14. The swimming pool analogy applied to the first mtpj - off balance. See Fig.1.12.

The abductor-adductor muscle balance is all important (Fig.1.12). The foot and its joints have muscles inside and outside the foot. The big toe has small muscles, and on the outer side (lateral), these are more powerful on the lateral side and comprise two strips, as shown. On the inner side (the arch side of the foot), the muscle is less powerful.

What is the function of the sesamoid bones, and why are they essential to foot mechanics?

The previous anatomical illustrations show bones marked as sesamoids (Figs. 1.9 & 1.11). The largest sesamoid in the body is the knee cap. The knee (patella) is a good example of maintaining the leg and thigh bone in alignment with the knee joint.

The first advice any physiotherapist and orthopaedic surgeon will give a knee sufferer is to keep the quadriceps (thigh muscles) strong. Sports podiatrist and dance specialist Simon Costain believes —

> Shoes are essential in and out of dance but restrict the movement and activity of muscles, so muscles become weaker. As a result, most dance injuries are caused by weak feet[6].

Theoretically, we can enhance the power of the abductor hallucis muscle, and indeed, some can. Not all toes are aligned in one direction. Those with a clear gap between the first and second toe have a straight toe, but occasionally, we see a toe in the opposite direction—hallux varus. Some people can move their toes from the second toe, but most create a downward pull unless the muscles have been trained along the lines Costain has suggested in dancers. Maintaining muscle power as we age is more challenging than retaining strength while young.

An idealistic image is shown of a method to strengthen the abductor muscle of the great toe. This does not mean pulling the toe over so as to hurt the foot, Fig.1.15. The toe is placed into the band and attempts are made to pull the band toward the middle between each foot against resistance.

---

[6] Costain, S. Specialising in Dance Podiatry— In Voices from Podiatric Medicine. Career Journeys Past & Present. Tollafield D R. Published by Busypencilcase Communications. 2023:P45

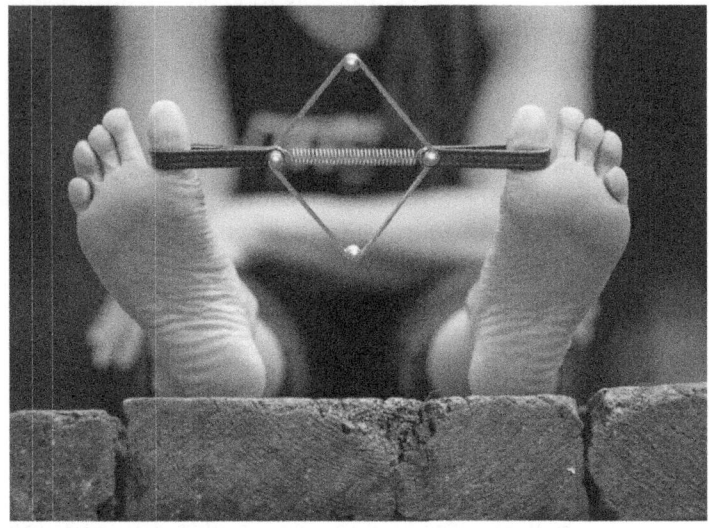

Fig.1.15. Strengthening the abductor muscles.

Two standard sesamoid bones act as pulleys. If you recall your school physics, a pulley is a wheel that allows a weight to be moved. The short flexor muscle-tendon (see Fig. 1.10) stabilises the proximal phalanx. If the sesamoid bone moves out of its pole position, the mechanical efficiency is lowered, and the muscle tendons on the lateral-outside (adductors) can create a sideways influence. X-rays allow us to assess the sesamoid apparatus and its relative position. The point of no return beyond the sesamoid is marked position 3, (Fig.1.15) bottom left in the X-ray picture. If that same bone moves to position 5, the alignment is beyond the point of no return. Consequently, the deformity fails to respond to conservative management.

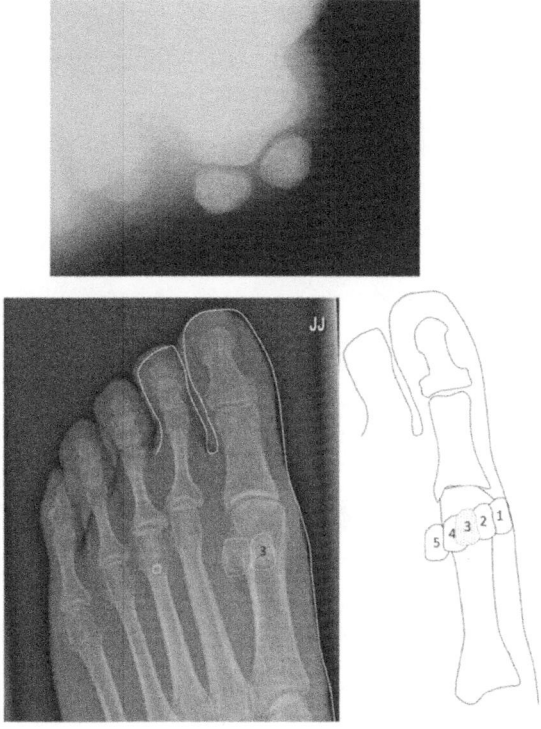

Fig.1.16. Sesamoid relationship with the first metatarsal.

Top – X-ray - normal sesamoid position where the seed like bones sit snuggly into the two grooves.

Bottom left — aligned with slight sesamoid displacement position. The small circle under the third metatarsal is a marker placed to show the position of a corn

Bottom right —drawing of different positions from 1 to 5. (Tollafield 2019)

Can a bump exist without the toe moving over?

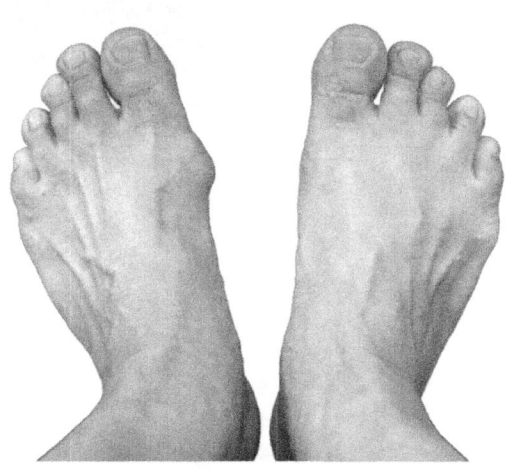

Fig.1.17. The left foot illustrates no hallux valgus, but a bump exists.

Where there is no hallux deviation, there are several possible causes. The most common feature is stiffness of the toe joint due to osteophyte formation. The bone overlies the joint, preventing movement. A stiff first toe joint is called hallux rigidus, derived from Latin. Osteophytes can arise on all sides of the mtpj. First-toe problems can arise due to stiff toes; however, where joints are affected by injury or inflammation, hallux valgus and bunion problems give rise to pain on weight-bearing. The mechanism described and illustrated in Fig.1.10 may no longer work. When the toe system of the purchase is less effective, pain can arise, and the muscles in the foot may be affected.

Joint Pathology

MTPJ open at surgery – head of the first metatarsal

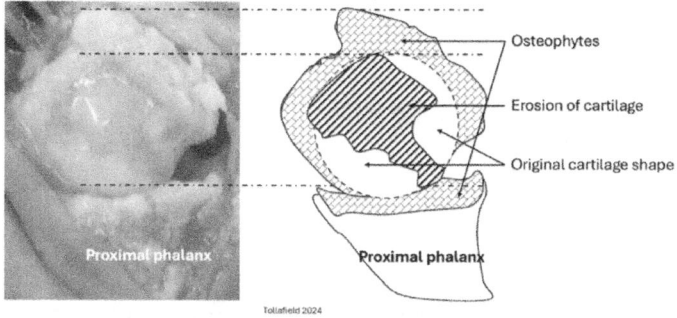

Fig.1.18. illustration showing osteophytes and cartilage damage.
(Tollafield 2024)

Injury can result from dropping a heavy weight on the foot or fracturing through the joint, metatarsal, or phalanges. Impact forces from stubbing the toe, whether against an object or as a result of sporting activities, cause inflammatory swelling, occasionally leading to permanent changes depending on the extent of internal joint damage.

The presence of an exostosis, which is only a way of saying excess bone, does not always limit the joint. As the joint enlarges—the two bones—the first metatarsal and proximal phalanx stop moving. Clinical examination will determine how much movement exists and if there is pain on movement. If worn over time, poorly fitting footwear, tight footwear, and damaged footwear linings will cause additional pressure on the side of the joint.

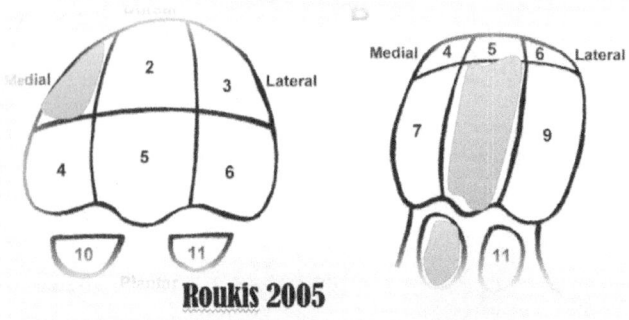

Fig.1.19. Roukis, 2005[7] recorded different locations split into defined areas. 1,8 and 10 proved most frequent.

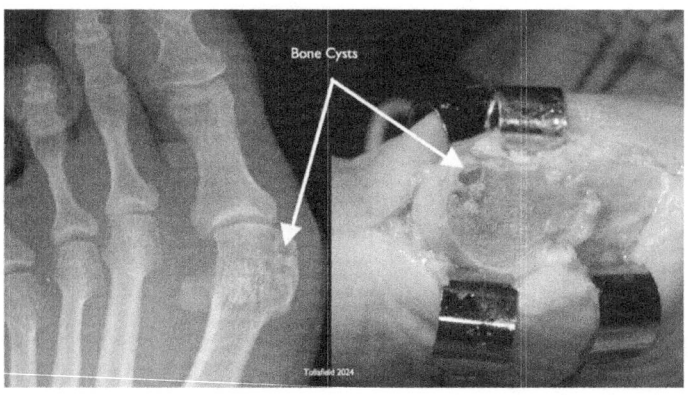

Fig.1.20. X-rays can highlight bone quality and aid the clinical diagnosis before surgery. However, X-rays do not show cartilage quality, and reliance on MRI is more valuable. (Tollafield 2024).

---

[7] Roukis, TS, Scott Weill, L Jn, Scott Weill, L Snr, Landsman, AS, Predicting articular erosion in hallux valgus: Clinical, radiographic and interoperative analysis. 2005;44,1:13-21

One of the curious problems of bone and joint damage is that even with extensive cartilage surface erosion, a patient may have few symptoms. There are several ways of analysing the joint without surgical intervention.

We can use X-rays or scans that take segmental sections, and the MRI scan offers one of the gold standards for diagnosis.

While the deformity may not be a concern, the direction of tendon pull will alter over time. A complete list of anatomical changes is outside the scope of this book, but suffice to say the anatomical relationship changes when a joint is repositioned.

Handouts, Information and Videos

Figure 1.20 represents a handout offered to patients but it is more than just information to be hidden away. As part of the consultations models, images, X-rays and written material should be explained. The original sheet was provided in colour to show different stages of cartilage change and joint loss.

The use of websites with images and pictorial information, including videos has started to improve patient consultations, especially where consent follows on.

As a generalisation the US produces more material on-line than the UK but much of it carries hard sell. However, there are some excellent sites in the UK produced by orthopaedic foot specialists. It is worth searching on-line for local specialist's websites.

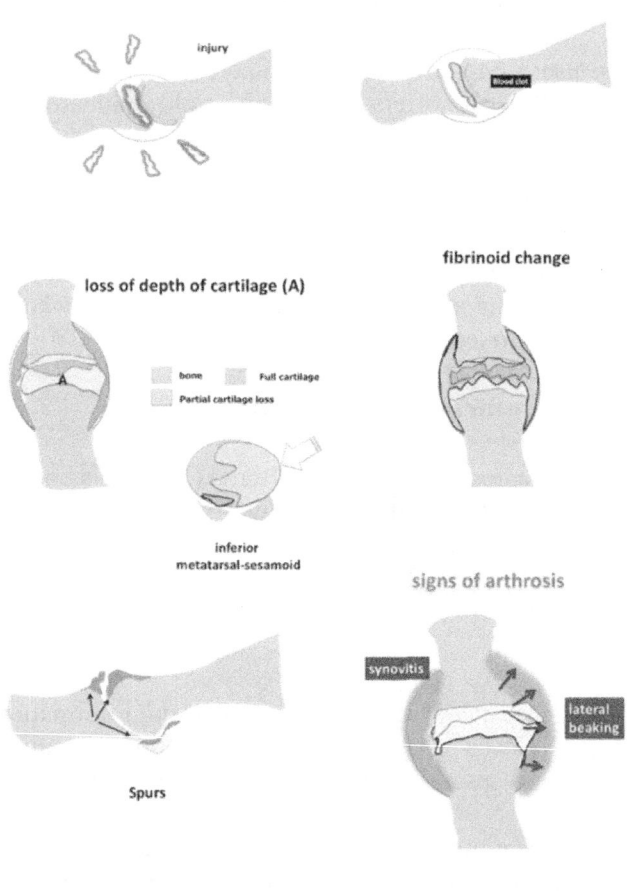

Fact sheet - Painful big toe. Changes associated with degeneration or arthritis.
© 2021Busypencilcase Communications for ConsultingFootPain

Fig.1.21. Illustrated patient information was provided to patients to explain the process behind arthrosis or degeneration leading to a stiff first toe. (Patient hand-out Tollafield 2021).

Posture and Gait

It may seem curious that a big toe could affect other body parts, but evidence suggests this is true.

CASE STUDY – Hip Pain

A lady wanted her hallux valgus corrected but also complained that her left hip was painful and causing problems. The surgery was duly performed, and when the time arrived for her final assessment, she burst into tears and explained that her hip pain had resolved after she had returned to regular walking. Anecdotal stories are easy to remember when successful treatment impacts general health.

A question often discussed between surgeons is whether the foot should be operated on before the knee. In our experience, knee surgeons are usually happy that the foot is operated first.

Because we compensate (make adjustments) to our body, both knees and hips will alter their movement as the forces produced by our weight and gravity exert muscle-tendon changes. The mechanics is not easy to understand. Fig 1.22. illustrates some alterations between weight bearing on both legs and feet and single leg-foot contact.

When the foot angles outwards or inwards, adapting for hallux valgus, the change depends on pain reduction, so we move our foot to toe-out.

If the toe joint is stiff, we tend to rotate the leg with the foot. The leg has to follow in a chain reaction upwards toward the hip and pelvis wherever the foot goes.

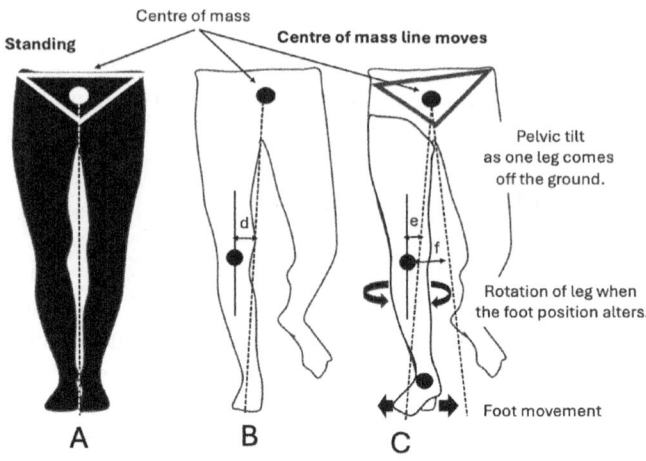

Fig.1.22. Centre of mass (effect of gravity on the lower limb and foot)[8]—adapted from Shi.

We have met the centre of mass shifting earlier with the swimming pool analogy and the body falling once the muscles can no longer overcome gravity.

A- Standing on both feet- the line from the centre of mass falls between the feet.

B- The left leg lifts to swing forward so the centre moves toward the foot, retaining ground contact.

C- As the foot moves, the leg rotates (curved arrows), causing another shift in the centre of mass (dotted line). As the foot moves in, the line moves out, and in the opposite case where the foot moves out, the line moves in.

---

[8] Shi, KS, Chien, HL, Lu, TW, Chang, CF. Gait changes in individuals with bilateral hallux valgus reduce first metatarsophalangeal loading but increase knee abductor moments. Gait & Posture. 40(2014)38-42

Additional effects include the pelvis and hip movement to compensate for the non-weight-bearing foot. Each joint has a centre, as the black or white circle shows. The knee circle shows the centre of mass moving close or further away, forcing muscles to work harder on one side.

These are the principles of biomechanics, but the reader only has to appreciate the changes in posture affect muscles elsewhere in the skeletal system.

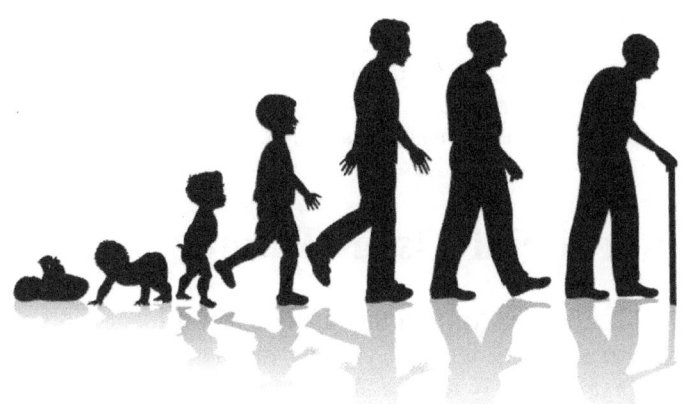

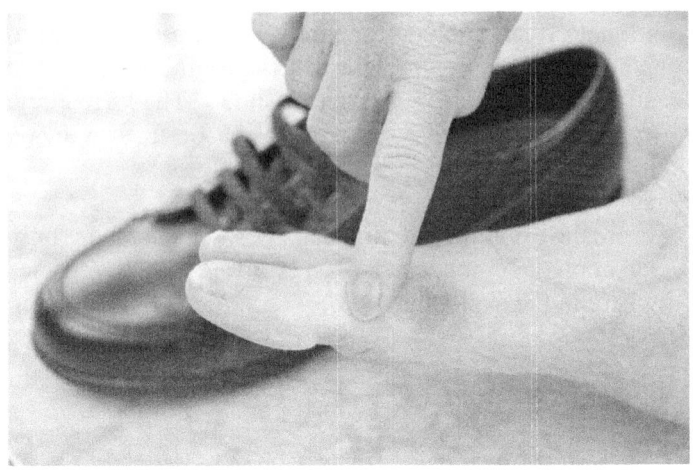

Fig.1.23. Exostosis on the side and top of the joint due to excessive bone deposits caused by long-standing pressure, inflammation, and damage. This is only sometimes due to shoes but may arise from injury and gout.

Superficial Tissue Damage

Skin can be rubbed from the outside, the inside, or in both directions. Our body has various mechanisms of coping. The first change is for the skin to form a blister. Next, we will see skin thickness increase (callus formation). Corns may form at the point of maximum pressure.

The skin may suffer chilling effects or even chilblains as we age because the local circulation is under pressure. While these are local to the top or side of the foot, careful footwear selection is vital. Select soft, deforming materials, ideally with no lining so that the leather will stretch over the bump. If you look at people's shoes, often the deformation of the shoe is the giveaway presence of hallux valgus or exostosis.

Ulceration & Deeper Damage

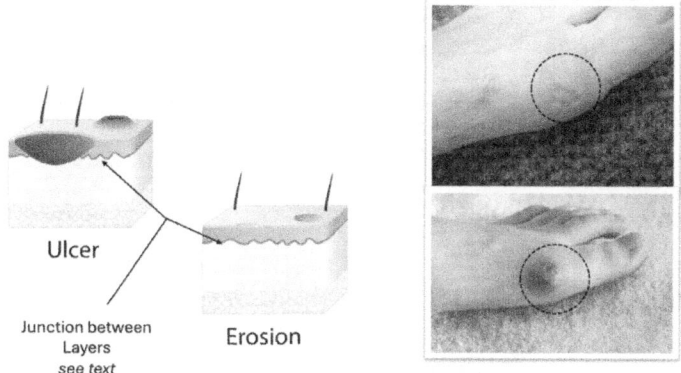

First metatarsophalangeal joint

Fig.1.24. Ulcer versus erosion. An adhesive pad has protected the first mtpj. Top right – erosion. Bottom right – pre-ulcerative skin breakdown. (Adapted Shutterstock +Tollafield 2024).

Ulceration is a deeper wound that may not heal. Unlike the erosive lesion, an ulcer can penetrate deeper than the junction between the upper and lower levels of the skin surface. Bleeding arises more readily once this junction has been breached. Poor circulation, infection, diabetes, and any condition leading to loss of sensation are concerns that should be dealt with by a professional.

The skin over the bunion is not the only location for changes—pressure changes can also cause pain in between the toes, under the ball of the foot, and in the hallux.

When the skin experiences constant pressure, callus and corn formation arise.

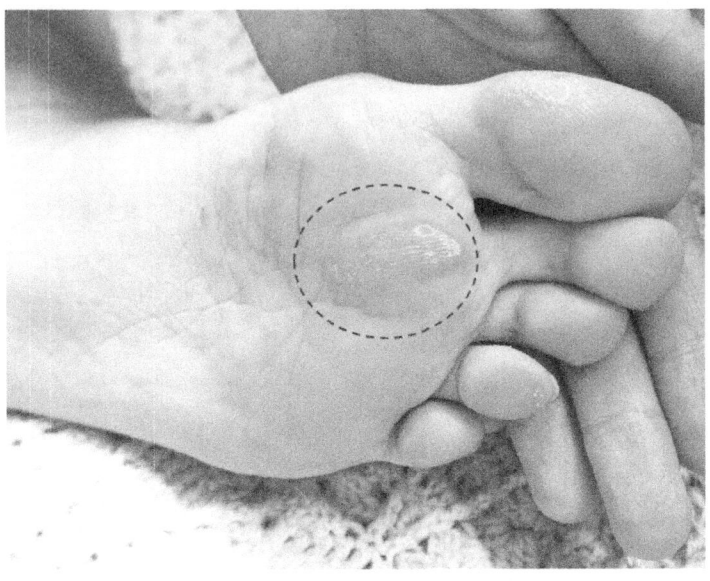

Fig.1.25. The pressure from altering the toe position may cause callus (circled) formation under the ball of the foot (second metatarsal) and inside of the great toe. Additionally, any of the smaller toes may be affected.

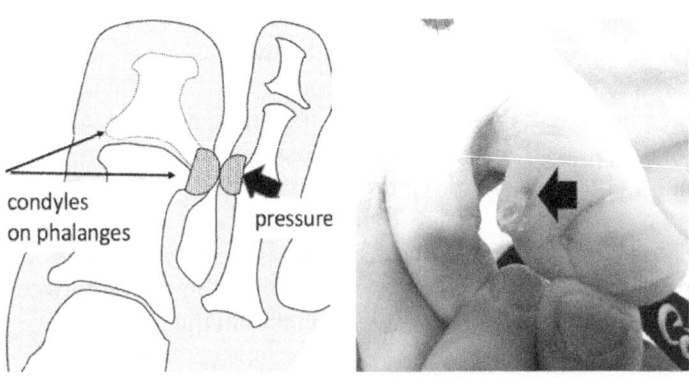

Fig.1.26. First and second toes with two bony condyles pressing on the skin in between toes can lead to callus, corns, blisters, erosions and ulcerations. (Tollafield 2024)

As the hallux drifts, it will influence the next toe, and a tight shoe will worsen the condition. See Fig.1.26, which shows bones pressing against the skin from inside.

Hallux valgus deformity can have far-reaching effects on foot pain, skin condition, footwear fit and comfort.

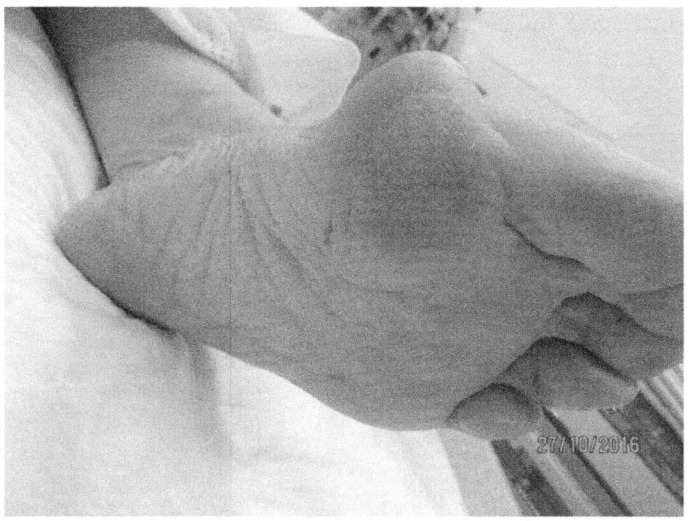

Fig.1.27. Skin pressure causes callus formation alongside the inside of the toe joint and contact surfaces. (Tollafield 2016)

Podiatrists specialise in managing changes in the skin associated with the deformity of hallux valgus and hammer toes.

Neuritic Bunion

A lesser-known problem, the neuritic bunion, is associated with hallux valgus deformity, where a superficial nerve branch runs over the mtpj and the bunion. If this is not managed, the nerve can thicken.

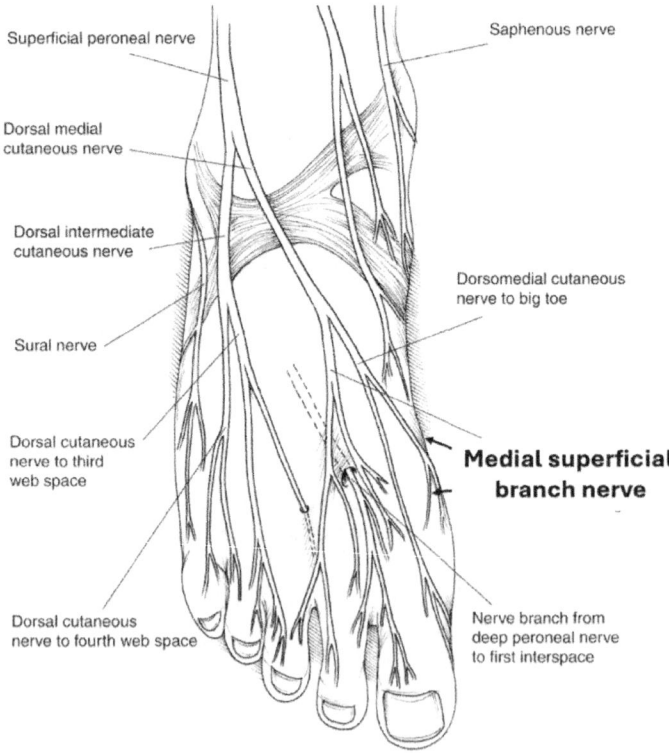

Superficial peroneal nerve

Saphenous nerve

Dorsal medial cutaneous nerve

Dorsal intermediate cutaneous nerve

Dorsomedial cutaneous nerve to big toe

Sural nerve

Dorsal cutaneous nerve to third web space

Medial superficial branch nerve

Dorsal cutaneous nerve to fourth web space

Nerve branch from deep peroneal nerve to first interspace

Fig.1.28. Medial superficial branch nerve. The illustration shows the complex nerve motorway on top of the foot. A branch runs over the first metatarsophalangeal joint, where the bone enlarges. (Courtesy MedicineBTG.com 2015. Permission 2024)

Once damaged, a nerve forms a swelling known as a neuroma. The locality of pain and tingling (paraesthesiae) suggests nerve involvement.

Hallux valgus does not need surgery if the nerve can be protected, and this is an area where self-help and conservative care can be valuable.

Persistent nerve pain can be responded to by reducing the exostosis or by relocating the branch and burying it. The frequency of neuritic bunion is low.

CASE STUDY – Nerve Damage

Upon exploration at surgery, a nerve appeared thickened and was removed as part of the superficial branch. The consistency was thickened and stiffer than the nerve's usual flexible, soft appearance. Numbness is expected but not always a problem if the pain can be resolved.

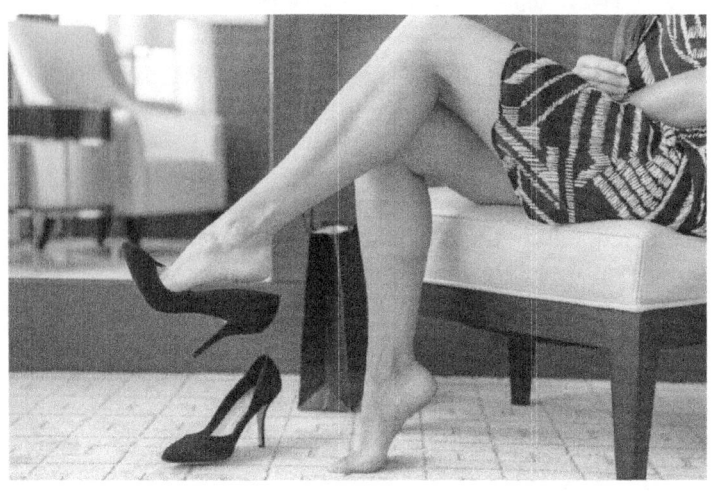

Causes Behind Hallux Valgus

Shoes do not cause hallux valgus, but footwear can result in bunion pain and provoke symptoms. While the most common question is what causes bunions (hallux valgus), the second question is whether we can prevent the deformity from arising. The simple answer is no, so we must manage hallux valgus. This reminds the reader of the difference between a bunion and a hallux valgus. We can mitigate the effect of some bunions if we understand the cause.

How Do You Get A Bunion?

No one could ask every living person if they had a bunion. The next best thing is to take a population sample, which does not rule out bias from country to country.

A research system called meta-analysis is considered valid and popular because it covers many published papers and accumulates information or data but is not itself the primary research.

Sheree Nix, (2010)[9] looked at seventy-six surveys in her meta-analysis, covering nearly half a million participants, and concluded that in adults (18–65 years of age), there was a 23% incidence of hallux valgus, this increased to nearly 38% in those aged 65+. This statistic shows that the extent of the deformity, judged by the angle of deviation, increases over our lives as we age. The distribution between men and women suggested a 13% and 30% bunion occurrence rate, respectively. This means women have twice the risk of having a bunion/HV condition.

Hannan and associates (2013)[10] state that:—

>...Hallux valgus and lesser toes are highly heritable in white men and women of European descent...

The study included over two thousand participants aged between 39-99. In a study in Nigeria prevalence in a black community was reported[11]. The study considered questionnaires from 979 returned respondents. The age covered 11-40. Interestingly, those affected with hallux valgus were 43.6% of males against the incidence of 56.4% of females.

---

[9] Nix, S, Smith, M, Vincenzino, B, Prevalence of hallux valgus in the general population: a systematic review and meta-analysis. 2010 https://doi.org/10.1186/1757-1146-3-21

[10] Hannan MT, Menz, HB, Jordan, JM, Cupples, LA, Cheng C-H, Hsu, Y-H. High Heritability of Hallux Valgus and Lesser Toe Deformities in Adult Men and Women. Arthritis Care & Research. 201.:65,9:1515-1521

[11] Akinbo SRA, Aiyegbusi AL, Owoeye OBA, Ogunsola MO. Prevalence of Hallux Valgus and related foot problems among individuals between the ages of 11 and 40 years. Nigerian Postgraduate Medical Journal 2011.18(1):51-55

The deformity worsened from 31-35 (given the highest age was 40)—thirty-four per cent presented with pain.

The importance of representing ethical groups cannot be understated. In contrast, Fig.1.29 shows a Caucasian mother and daughter side by side with the same deformity, and yet there are other cases where a grandmother and granddaughter have the condition, where the generation in between (the mother) is missed out.

Root, Weed & Orien (1977)[12] show a picture of a proud male African native standing for a photo. He had never worn shoes, and yet he had a severe bunion. Poor footwear can aggravate a deformity and reveal problems across the whole forefoot. Shoes do not cause bunions; evidence arises from multiple sources.

The mystery of the origins of the bunion leaves us to suspect that the features of hallux valgus lie within our human (genetic) makeup. More women come forward than men, but the gender bias may be distorted by footwear, vanity and women's tendency to visit healthcare professionals more than men.

---

[12] Root, M, Orien, WP, Weed, JH Normal and Abnormal Function. Clinical Biomechanics Volume II. Clinical Biomechanics Corporation. 1977.P386 Fig.10.41.

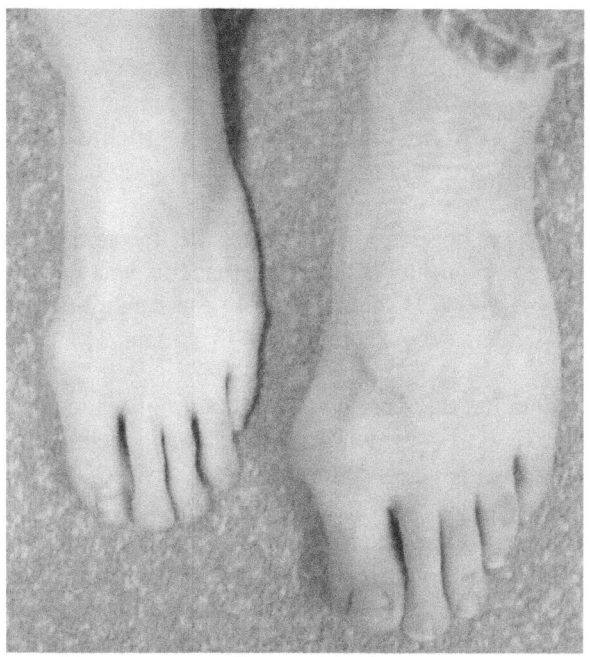

Fig.1.29. Mother and daughter compare deformity, which interestingly shows on the same side. The daughter (left-side foot) also has a small tailor's bunion, the equivalent bunion affecting the fifth toe. (Tollafield 2019)

Timeline[13]

A good example of the cause and effect of hallux valgus can be seen in dancers or athletes when they are young. Damage sustained in youth can creep into later life. The phenomenon of a timeline is important to understand. The simplest way of describing this can be related to the extent of internal joint damage.

---

[13] Tollafield, DR, Injury & Timeline in Foot Health Myths, Facts & Fables. Podiatry Reflections. Busypencilcase Communications. 2021:22-25

Once irreparable, the joint will continue to deteriorate, and the golden period to resolve problems will narrow. Successful treatment will depend on timeline factors as established joint damage is more challenging to remedy.

'Turf toe' can be seen in field sports, but the same effect can arise in, for example, dancers; earlier, this was described as an impact injury. Because of footwear constraints (lack of room), dancers favour taping and dressings.

While dancing does not cause hallux valgus, the symptoms associated with a growing deformity and deterioration of cartilage can create joint inflammation with soft tissue tears.

There is insufficient evidence to demonstrate conclusively that dancing, specifically pointe work, increases the prevalence or severity of hallux valgus; more research is needed. Treatment of hallux valgus in dancers should be conservative, with a delay of surgical correction until retirement if possible. (Davenport, K, 2014)[14].

---

[14] Davenport, Kathleen & Simmel, Liane & Kadel, Nancy. (2014). Hallux Valgus in Dancers: A Closer Look at Dance Technique and Its Impact on Dancers' Feet Journal of Dance Medicine & Science 18(2) DOI: 10.12678/1089-313X.18.2.86

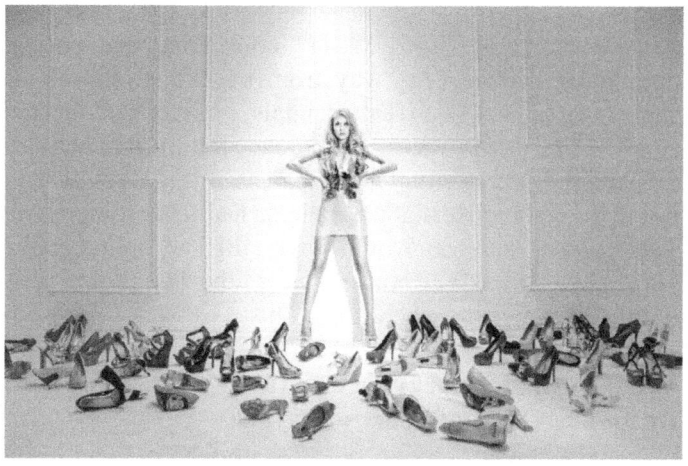

Fig. 1.30. Footwear has traditionally been considered a leading cause of hallux valgus.

Footwear As A Cause Of Bunions

Few studies examine multiple risk factors for hallux valgus, although Nguyen (2010)[15] considered a study involving a sample of community-dwelling older women and men in the USA. One of the study's conclusions reflected the biological, structural, and behavioural differences in men and women. This means we respond differently in our cellular bodies and how we act out in life, both in dress code and attitude to intersocial relationships. Nguyen considered that gender imposed different factors, borne out by twice the number of females to men that suffer. The relationship between body weight and height (body mass index, BMI), high-heeled shoes, and flat feet is all associated with foot pain in the presence of HV.

[15] Nguyen US, Hillstrom, HJ, et al. Factors Associated With Hallux Valgus In A Population-Based Study Of Older Women And Men. Osteoarthritis. 2010;18(1):41-86

A Japanese study (Kato 1981)[16] considered that once the population had moved away from traditional shoe styles, such as Geta socks and Tabi sandals, in favour of Western-style shoes, orthopaedic surgeons found an increased demand for operations. The weakness of this study was that it failed to recognise that the patients had few problems with Tabi sandals and yet would have still had hallux valgus. Once they used Western footwear, the symptoms arose, unlike the condition of hallux valgus.

What Other Researchers Have Said About The Influence Of Footwear

Piqué-Vidal (2007)[17] reviewed 350 subjects across three generations. The ratio of women to men with bunions was nearly 15:1, providing a genetic line of argument as a 56% likelihood. The female sex predominated with regard to the gender of parents with *hallux valgus* ... (the) severity of *hallux valgus* was not significantly influenced by gender, the affected branch of the family, or gender of the affected relatives. Family history of bunion deformity was present in 90% ... affecting some family members across three generations, which is compatible with autosomal dominant inheritance with incomplete penetrance.

The incidence of HV deformity in Iranian university students, as a sample of Iranian youngsters, is much higher than those in some Western societies. This deformity was shown to be highly inherent due to the increasing level of this deformity among first-degree relatives.

---

[16] Kato, T, Watanabe, S The Etiology of Hallux Valgus in Japan. Clin. Orthop. & Rel. Res. 1981;157:78-81

[17] Piqué-Vidal, C, Sole, MT, Antich, J. Hallux Valgus Inheritance Pedigree Research In 350 Patients With Bunion Deformity. J. Foot & Ankle Surg. 2007;46(3)149-165

Routine use of high-heel or round-tip shoes showed no influence on the rate of HV deformity. Abbas Rahimi et al. (2012)[18]

Risk factors for hallux valgus… may include increasing age, female gender, genetic predisposition, constrictive shoe wear, first-ray hypermobility, foot architecture, tight Achilles' tendon, and first metatarsal length. Davenport et al. (2014)[9].

Can pregnancy cause a Hallux valgus?

When pregnant, the hormones can also loosen joints throughout the body to prepare for childbirth by softening the pelvis. The foot is not excluded, and increased deformity may arise following pregnancy.

The centre of mass alters in pregnancy as the foetus affects the pelvis and will also influence hip, knee and foot. Fig. 1.21. offers some of the basic principles in changing postural biomechanics.

Do health conditions cause bunions?

Neuromuscular conditions and rheumatoid arthritis can cause bunions. Muscle and tendon imbalance may prevail in nerve-related conditions, which may be genetic.

Rheumatoid arthritis can cause joint breakdown and destroy essential joint anatomy, including bone density. Albeit rare, treatment for this inflammatory disease is better understood and treated today.

---

[18] Rahimi, A, Rezaee M, Behrouzi, R Maemi, S. Incidence Of Hallux Valgus Deformity Among Iranian Students. Tibb-I Tavanbakhshi. 2021;1(2):45052

Flat feet can influence foot mechanics, but this condition does not automatically lead to hallux valgus.

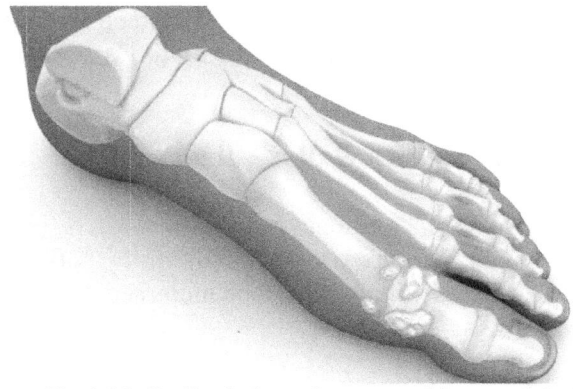

Fig.1.31. Stylised view of gouty tophi around the joint

Gout does not cause a bunion. It is the product of abnormal chemistry that deposits crystals or urate in the joint lining. It is destructive, painful, and prevents movement. An existing hallux valgus deformity may be involved with gout's features producing stiffness once the cartilage has been destroyed.

Part I - Summary

A bunion is a bump, and hallux valgus is a deformity that can be minor, moderate, or severe and affect other toes.

The bump is called an exostosis if bony but may have a cyst associated with a ganglion or bursa.

The first toe's anatomy comprises several joints comprising two phalanges and a metatarsal. The first toe joint is known as the first metatarso-phalangeal joint or mtpj.

Two tiny round bones, called sesamoids, exist under the first metatarsal and act as a pulley, ensuring the toe is stable when the heel lifts.

The sesamoids drift out of alignment in hallux valgus because the first and second metatarsals start to play. If the toe rotates with the deformity, more pressure is placed on the nail groove.

Faulty mechanical alignment adds to joint wear and tear and altered foot position against the leg and knee.

Pain can arise in the knee and hip as the knee rotation alters the muscles above the knee.

The cause of hallux valgus appears hereditary and affects more women than men across all ethnic groups. Footwear adds to the symptoms but not the cause. Hallux valgus can skip a generation.

Hallux valgo-rigidus arises with joint stiffening and may relate to injury. Joint pain may drive a person to seek urgent treatment. Once rigid, the toe tends to remain in that position. Not all rigid toes are painful.

Osteophytes are excessive bone projections around joints and limit movement.

While many toes have a mild valgus position (less then 5-15°, some are straight, and others may have a varus position.

The skin around the first mtpj is at risk from pressure with poor circulation and numbness.

Progressive hallux valgus is more prevalent from age 35 upwards. Young people can suffer marked hallux valgus, but early surgical intervention should be avoided.

Part II

Since hallux valgus provokes the question of footwear fit and comfort, many methods exist to alleviate the main concerns.

Dividing the options into self-help—what you can do to assist yourself and when to seek advice forms the main objective behind Part II.

Self-help

We have anticipated that this section may be more important to some people, especially those who have heard bad stories about surgery, those frightened about the prospects of 'going under the knife' or simply going into hospital. Because such stories about a family member or friend having a bad experience, it is not unreasonable that phobia grows. The big question is, *what can I do to help myself?* To apply helpful self-help techniques, it is important to understand the big toe joint and some of the problems associated with the deformity.

Misleading Information

Trawling published lay titles such as *Bye Bunions: A Guide for Dancers, The Hallux Valgus Cure – Natural Method and Fixing Bunions Without Surgery* are not unattractive[19]. Any title that draws consumers to believe bunions can be 'fixed' stretches the truth. The inference that the deformity can be cured with non surgical methods is not possible.

---

[19] Such titles are real, misleading, badly produced and should be avoided.

Can bunions be made more comfortable?

This section concentrates on deciding what you need: advice versus pain management. There are several things you can do yourself, but you should only continue with self-treatment if matters improve. You should wait no longer than 48 hours if the pain is due to infection or potential fracture or if your diabetes becomes unstable in the presence of a skin problem.

Reasons To Consider Treatment

No one should be pushed into making surgical decisions, but it helps to understand what can arise without appropriate management; so, if you have jumped Part I, consider the following:-

---

Do I have a painful bump?
Is my toe joint painful?
Does my toe cross and push my second or third toes out of alignment?
Do I have shoe fitting problems?
Is my foot unsightly—I hate going to the beach.
Is it that I don't want my foot to become worse?
Am I plagued with corn and hard skin?

Having read the first pages of this book, you should know how to make your diagnosis. The second concern is when to seek help and how much you can help yourself. We know that hallux valgus may involve a prominence.

As long as the bump receives no excessive pressure, the skin will cope, and the fluid-like cysts that form a ganglion or bursa will not worsen.

Do I need to do something?
If I need to have something done, can I avoid surgery?
If surgery is necessary, what does it involve?
How would surgery affect me?

Careful Selection of Footwear

Check for damage to the lining inside the shoe prevent skin irritation at the joint level. A prominent joint will cause the shoe's lining to tear over time, damaging the skin. Avoid second-hand shoes that are damaged, and generally avoid second hand altogether where possible. Allow for wider shoes to accommodate the width. The best upper material allows stretching.

How can we protect the skin?

First, we must look at the shoe. Ideally, it must have three properties: It must fit a widening foot. Ensure a new-fitting shoe is adopted before pressure builds, especially if the big toe drifts. If a second toe lies on top of the hallux, the depth of the shoe becomes critical as you will have two points that rub. Select a shoe that fits the wider foot and use an insock for the smaller foot. Width is the main issue.

Here are two links. <u>Healthy feet store</u>[20] in the UK and <u>Ability Hacker</u>[21] in the US provide some advice for different-size shoe

purchases. While these are not recommendations, they illustrate the opportunity to fit feet with different sizes in the same style. We wish to remind you that using these links can be withdrawn or fail, so you may need to seek out similar options.

Stretching The Material

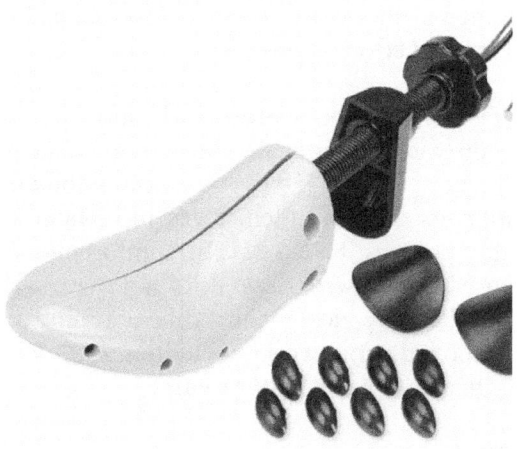

Fig.2.1. The <u>shoe tree</u>[22] has small holes to insert stretching buttons. Several designs are available and can be purchased from reputable sources on the internet.

---

[20] Healthy feet store.
https://www.healthyfeetstore.com/collections/bunion-shoes-for-women-and-men-bunion-footwear

[21] https://www.abilityhacker.com/where-to-buy-shoes-when-your-feet-are-two-different-sizes/

[22]https://video.search.yahoo.com/search/video?fr=aaplw&ei=utf-8&p=stretching+your+shoe+to+make+it+bigger#action=view&id=3&vid=1839c432f3604b76c8b2526e8a7b58da

You can take a shoe that fits closely but needs to be stretched. Some cobblers will provide this service, but for the most part, stretching the shoe using newspaper forced into the end will help and is cheap. The shoe tree is best for stretching specific points, such as the top and side of the shoe. Fig.2.1 shows an example of a brand; this is available to purchase from £15.00[23] upwards.

If stretching solves the problem, investing in a shoe tree made from wood is probably best. The problem arises if the shoe material is plastic or has a non-yielding lining. It comes down to selecting suitable footwear material. Leather is still one of the best materials; if the inside is rough, it will stretch better. Women's shoes are slightly less adaptable than traditional men's Oxford styles.

Footwear fashion will be a problem if surgery is not an option. If you wear fashionable shoes, remember to wear them for the shortest time. If they are essential for work, and today, employers can find themselves in difficulties with rigid clothing policies, take a pair of comfortable shoes to change into when footwear style does not matter. Sandals and open-toe shoes are ideal in the right environment, which brings us to the industrial working environment, where risk from injury becomes part of your routine.

Different workplaces, from shops to factories, may have policies affecting men and women regarding required footwear. Health and Safety was enforced in 1974 in the UK. The significant feature is the need for the employer to look after the employee's welfare, which means foot protection in at-risk environments. While your firm might provide protective shoes with steel toe caps, not all shoes and boots are suited to foot problems.

---

[23] Prices stated are quoted as at 2024.

Discuss this with your firm before accepting footwear, and also ask if you can use different grades of shoes that still provide protection but can avoid pressure of the enlarged toe joint.

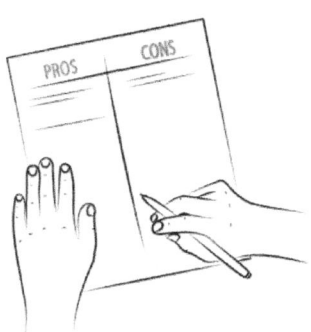

Protecting The Joint

Protecting your bunion with wise shoe selection and stretching alone may fix the problem. Occasionally, you will need surface protection.

Felt and foam adhesive materials can be shaped and formed to protect the skin. Local protection using a felt dressing is discussed with the support in this six-minute **video**[24], produced for this book. The pad with adhesive backing will act as a first-aid dressing.

YouTube · David Tollafield
370+ views · 5 years ago   ⋮

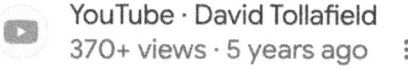
How to make a bunion pad

---

[24] https://www.youtube.com/watch?v=GCVmipZPq6M

For this book use YouTube as above.

Cut out a small cavity in the material without going through the full thickness of felt on the adhesive side. Leave enough sticky material to contact the skin. Only use felt once broken skin has healed and strengthened. As emphasised in the video, some warnings exist when using adhesive-backed dressings. Use semi-compressed felt bought online or from a pharmacy outlet to make your dressing. Felt is perfect because it moulds around the deformed area, bedding down to provide comfort within shoes.

Foam does not mould around the joint as well as felt. Ensure you have the correct location. Use for 1-2 days only. These dressings can slip if not applied as shown.

Avoid continuous use. If you retain the adhesive for over a few days, you risk skin damage.

Avoid damaged and infected skin, where the foot has no sensation, chilblains and skin with poor circulation. Never reapply a dressing, especially if it becomes wet. If the pad becomes wet, replace it with a fresh dressing pad.

The use of adhesive material has been surpassed by the advent of gel-like dressings, often made from rubberised silicone. Plastic technology has advanced, making products accessible to patients and those with foot problems. Bunion sleeves or shields are now available from high street pharmacies and online.

The material must be thin enough to fit inside a shoe and firmly on the foot to avoid slippage. The image shown over the page— Fig.2.2 includes a small interdigital wedge in the right hand image.

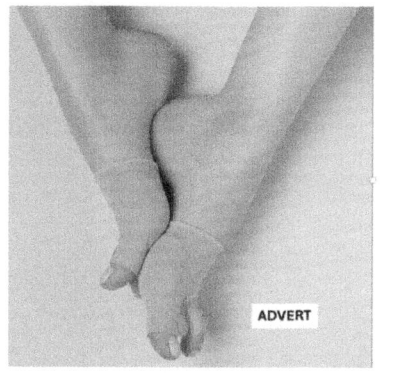 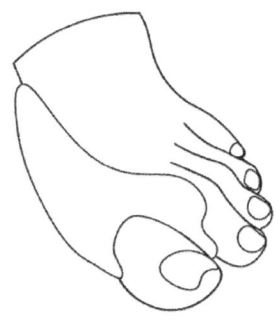

Fig.2.2. Bunion shield or sleeve

There are many designs of bunion shields on the market, but we can only provide a guide to selection. If you are uncomfortable with a wedge between the toes, select a design without a wedge. If you have corns interposing against those condylar prominences, a soft wedge protects against skin rub.

First Aid

When skin blisters become infected, an antiseptic cream after washing with boiled water left to cool can be used or a sterile pack of normal saline (salty water). The latter product comes in 25ml sachets (Fig.2.3). An adhesive sterile dressing-type plaster with a pad is helpful in the early stages of wound protection and, if left off at night, enhances healing once any sign of discharge has cleared.

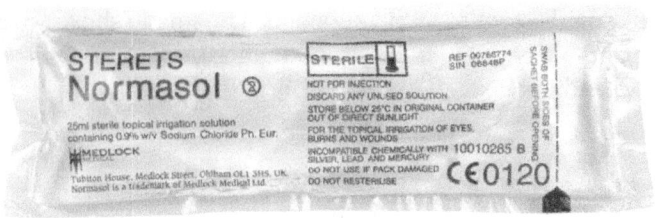

Fig.2.3. A convenient solution for instant sterile cleaning of open wounds

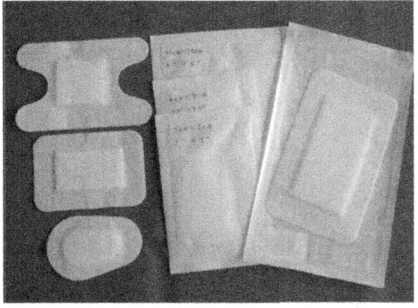

Fig.2.4. Shaped dressings are worth considering unless you are creative with sharp scissors.

Adhesive dressings should be retained in prepacked sterile condition ready for use. The material shown in Fig.2.4 is lighter than the former zinc oxide fabric. The butterfly (top left) is helpful for toes.

Antiseptics

When combatting or preventing wound weeping (infection), povidone-iodine and chlorhexidine creams and ointments are preferred over antibiotic creams. If in doubt, seek a pharmacist's advice.

Chilblains

Broken chilblains need to be treated like wounds, but when not broken, ensure correct footwear and insulation against cold and dampness. Footwear should be loose rather than tight, so too many socks are not ideal. Chilblains do not focus on age alone; younger people still suffer from progressive hallux valgus, although hallux valgus generally deteriorates as we age. The youngest sufferer the authors have seen is a nine-year-old with a deformity as large as her grandmother's bunion.

Skin damage

Dry skin or cracks (fissures) benefit from regular cream application. Many hand creams play the same role and may prove less expensive. Barrier creams afford better water-repellent action, but daily application rubbed well into the skin improves skin texture and strength.

Pain Management

Pain should subside once wounds are made comfortable, but standard household cabinet medication such as paracetamol (acetaminophen—US) or ibuprofen is helpful. Pain not alleviated may benefit from professional help. Analgesic tablets are designed to assist pain until healing follows. The standard guideline in the UK is to seek professional help if, after 2-3 days, pain does not subsist.

Cyst & Bunions

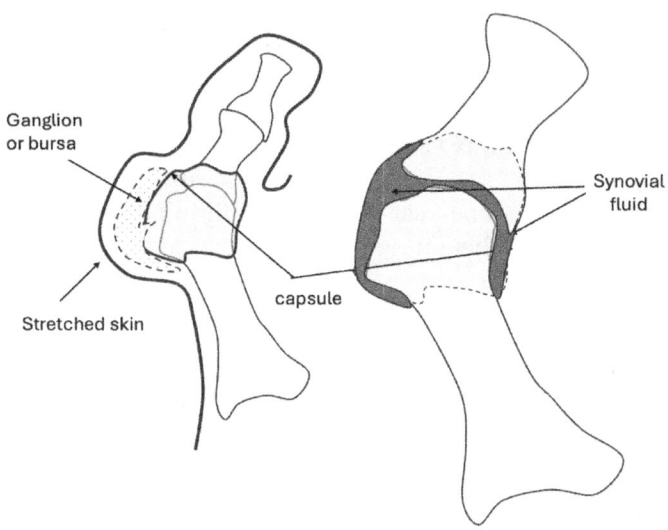

Ganglion
or bursa

Synovial
fluid

Stretched skin

capsule

Fig.2.5. The bunion arises with deeper pressure damage affecting
the joint lining.

We can refer to ganglia and bursae as cysts (Fig.2.5). Earlier, we discussed the deeper part of the skin forming fluid. This becomes obvious if you press your finger down onto the skin, where an indentation returns when pressure is released. This spongy material relates to an organised sac filled with a clear sticky gel or fluid.

The joint is made up of a capsule—this is a sheath-like structure reinforced with fibres for strength, Fig.2.5. A synovial membrane produces special joint fluid upon which healthy cartilage is maintained in optimum condition and the two ends of the mtpj glide. If the capsule is damaged, the lining protrudes and leaks, forming an outer membrane.

The ganglion has a thin gossamer lining, while the bursa is more organised and has a thicker lining.

Is it true you can make a ganglion disappear?

Ganglions (plural - ganglia) can shrink without treatment, but bursae tend not to collapse and retain their spongy pouch. The pathology is complex and is beyond further discussion in this book, but such swellings can be inconvenient.

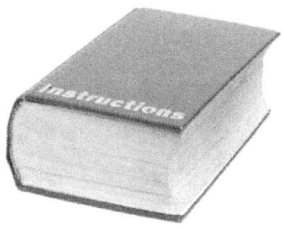

Fig.2.6. A heavy book is not the answer for cystic swellings.

You might be persuaded to hit this with a book. The Bible[25] often represented an accessible book and had nothing to do with religion. While there are plenty of sources of heavy books, any form of forced hitting tissue is not recommended, and indeed, one should avoid using computer tablets and iPads in place of the Bible - that is, unless you are searching for information!

---

[25] As the anecdotes came from a time when the UK was predominantly Christian, other representative religious groups were not mentioned as in the Koran (Qur'an – Moslem), Torah (Judaism), Tipitaka (Buddhism) or books (poems) used by Hindus.

We have seen ganglions arise over the top of the foot; sometimes, these can even be associated with the main toe tendon. Tears are so small that you cannot detect them on ultrasound unless the fluid and its lining are large, forming the catch-all term - cyst. Just because you may have cysts elsewhere in the body does not imply any relationship with the ganglionic cyst, sometimes known as a synovial cyst. The impact of a heavy book on a ganglion will reduce the swelling, as the thin lining will collapse, but the membrane lining can reform. Ganglionic cysts become a nuisance in tight shoes that press against bone. They occur commonly with big toe deformity (hallux valgus). Scans such as MRIs can help determine the extent of involvement.

Ganglia are the most common form of cysts on the medial side of the first mtpj. Bursae are more commonly found under the foot.

Taping

You can reduce the impact of soft tissue swelling by selecting the most appropriate footwear, from open-toe shoes to broader, soft, stretchy materials.

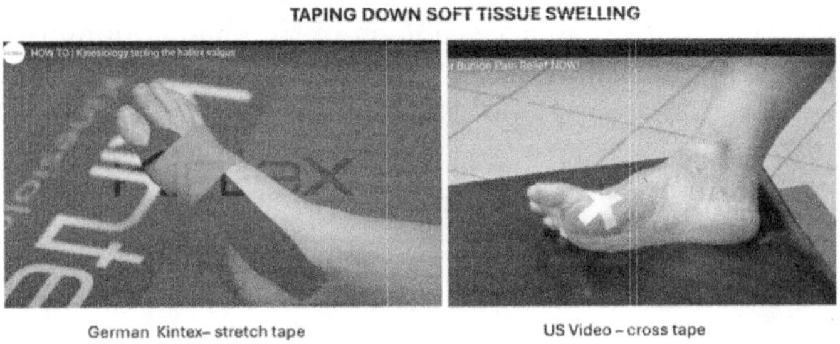

TAPING DOWN SOFT TISSUE SWELLING

German Kintex– stretch tape   US Video – cross tape

Fig.2.7. Two Videos on YouTube. Links are shown in the footnote.

In acute, or painful periods where the skin is intact, a thin dressing that tapes the swelling so it does not move can protect the skin. Some links are provided using simple methods with rigid strapping and the newer Kinesio tapes. The strongest advice remains as with felt adhesive techniques—don't apply to damaged, weak or fragile skin, and always heal a wound with first aid before applying any tape. If diabetic and the disease is not stable, seek advice first from a professional. Never leave tape on for longer than two days, and do not reapply when the skin is moist from creams or bathing. If the skin becomes inflamed, stop applying tape.

The first suggestion from a US site (3.20m) uses a cross tape[26] and then binds the foot around the forefoot. In the second video, produced by Kintex[27], Germany, a stretchy material is used, hence the word *kinesio*. In this short video (1.53m), the tape will achieve the same objective as the US video.There are a wide variety of self-help videos, many of which are lengthy and of poor quality. We recommend shorter videos under seven minutes, avoiding those with a strong sales pitch. The painful bunion needs to be immobilised to settle inflammation. Use YouTube for the links below by name e.g Kintex. There are numerous, US made videos on taping for bunions. We have produced a short video (5.19m) using the fan strap technique[28].

---

[26]https://video.search.yahoo.com/search/video;_ylt=AwrFANewYs1m
MC4NGB77w8QF;_ylu=c2xrA3RleHQEaXQDQWxzb1RyeQRzZWM
DcmVsBHBvcwMy?p=B+Union+Tape&fr2=p:s,v:v,m:rs-
top,ct:relatedSearches&fr=aaplw#action=view&id=7&vid=57457d4c71
9cc22c7bc4be8db9e38764

[27]https://video.search.yahoo.com/search/video;_ylt=AwrFANewYs1m
MC4NGB77w8QF;_ylu=c2xrA3RleHQEaXQDQWxzb1RyeQRzZWM
DcmVsBHBvcwMy?p=B+Union+Tape&fr2=p:s,v:v,m:rs-
top,ct:relatedSearches&fr=aaplw#id=12&vid=8ffdfb0b9f54ae36ab6fa84
95099fb39&action=view

[28] https://www.youtube.com/watch?v=RwFeqCr0LQU&t=7s

Fig.2.8.— ideally, the tape should be 2.5cm wide and not stretchy. Six 10cm lengths should be cut and ends rounded to prevent peeling back. Tape can come on rolls or with backing. The tape is overlapped half and half, attached first to the toe end, and pulled under tension to adhere around the midfoot. There are many different methods of taping the first toe, but this is a tried and tested design that has been used for over 45 years. The illustration shows the fan strap below, which can be accessed using the link shown.

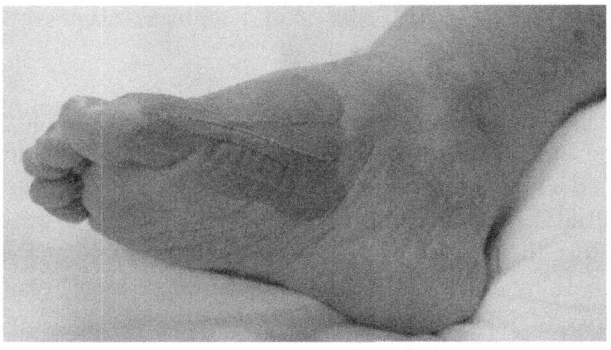

Fig.2.8. Fan Strapping limits pain and movement around the joint and assists swelling by compressing the fluid. (Tollafield 2020)

Splints & Spacers

First, there were books on how to exercise the bunion away, implying that you can stop genetic destiny. Now, there are a plethora of splints that, if used, will prevent the bunion from arising.

As scientists and avid researchers in foot health medicine, we prefer to follow the science. Patients often ask if the splint is valuable for their hallux valgus.

The splint has a purpose and function and might add value. The quick fix and its low cost are close to our hearts—while not a criticism it is how humans think. Splints replace the taping methods suggested above and can help with pain and reduce some of the muscle fatigue we refer to as spasms.

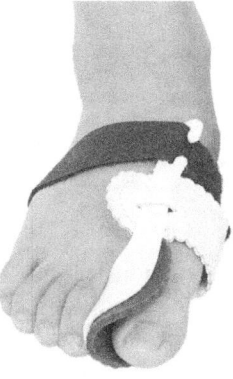

Fig.2.9. Rigid night splint. Softer forms may be better tolerated.

The big toe (hallux) splint is often called a 'night splint' (Fig 2.9), which implies that it can only be worn at night. In reality, many designs can be worn during the day. Both splints can assist the patient; there is no reason why one should not be used overnight and the other during the day. Rigid splints cannot be worn in closed shoes.

Spacers

The internet is littered with different modalities for sale, which are within reach of most pockets. Spacers are advocated because you can wedge soft rubber molds in between the first and second toe and the toe straightens. This does not correct the toe, but it does stop pressure between the bony prominences that occur.

Pressure can occur equally on the arch side of the big toe, resulting in a thickened skin ridge. In the latter case, it is not necessary to have hallux valgus. Dark areas within the callus suggest small bleeds within the skin. There should be of no concern, and the callus can be softened or reduced with a pumice stone or modern rotary shaver, now popular for hardened areas of skin.

Understanding the lining of the first toe joint

If we ignore the toe's position (the position of the valgus) and turn our focus to the joint, the 'splint' offers some assistance. We need to consider how and why a splint works.

A capsule surrounds the joint (Fig.2.5). The lining within the capsule produces fluid that nourishes the joint and cartilage. That lining has a rich blood supply. If the lining (synovium) swells, synovial fluid is added to the joint, which does less well. If blood arises within the joint, it forms mini clots that scar the joint and reduce movement. Normal joint fluid is clear and thin. An abnormal joint fluid changes colour and thickens. Nerves that supply the joint tell the brain the joint is swollen and painful. Nerves also tell the small muscles to tighten up, resulting in involuntary spasms that cause pain and limit joint movement as it stiffens. Of course, some of this stiffening is part of the protective mechanism. Over time, the cartilage lining the bone cracks, causing fissures and tears. Cartilage is essential for smooth gliding movements but can withstand more damage than we realise. If inflamed, the lining causes symptoms of movement. The night splint can assist in resting the joint, and taping or a daytime splint can limit painful movement during the day.

By holding the joint open, the inflammatory changes can be assisted. Chronic changes however may fair less well depending on the damage present. Forget the soft neoprene or latex splints that promise bunion correction, although they might be better than nothing. We need to look for something a little firmer, something with a plastic skeleton and adjustability. Sadly, all the products found online will use the word 'correcting bunions'—this will not happen, but the inflamed joint may calm down—and this is a good thing.

Use the splint to help recover from a painful toe. Strapping the toe can be helpful, but only for short periods because of skin irritation. Fan strapping is excellent for day use, but the night splint works better while at rest and saves the skin from irritation and potential sensitivity. Our video on joint manipulation shows a simple exercise[29] (3.04m).

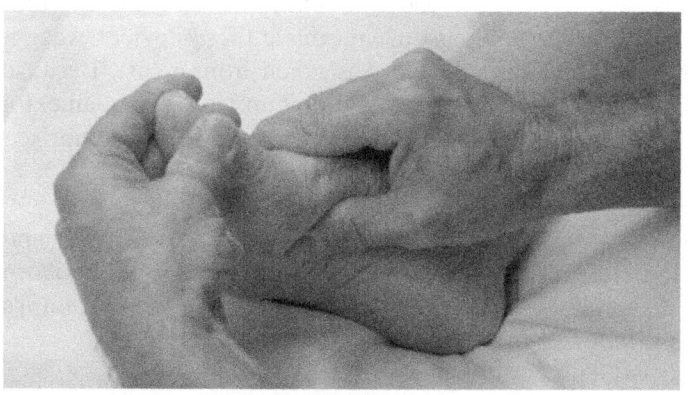

Fig.2.10. Exercise is important in assisting arthritic conditions by moving congestion and improving joint lubrication. (Tollafield 2019).

---

[29] https://www.youtube.com/watch?v=QIRm6r-yUSk&t=39s : Use *'youtube stiff and painful toe joint Tollafield'* for this book to search for the video.

Night splint combined with an insole

Ali Tehraninasar[30] examined thirty female patients aged 19-45 (2008). The research divided the women into two groups – one wore an insole with a toe separator, and the other wore a night splint. The period of follow-up was three months.

Pain was measured by intensity, a reference we call a visual analogue scale (VAS). The patient marks a 10cm line, and as pain becomes more intense, the mark is closer to the 10cm end than the 0cm end. The visual analogue pain scale is often used as a numerical scale of 1 to 5 or 1 to 10. The researcher used a 10 cm line.

Tehraninasar found the insole and toe separator had a better effect than the night splint when controlling pain. The insole was semi-rigid and ended behind the ball of the foot (metatarsals). The person who made these devices was an orthotist, and each device was taken from a cast. Because the material used in the design took up more room, an extra +1 shoe size was necessary. The night splint comprised moldable foam and a rigid polyethylene bar.

Splints are valuable in reducing pain and muscle spasms and can be useful after surgery. Most splints can only be worn without shoes, except the shields protecting the first mtpj's bony side.

---

[30] Tehraninasar, A, Saeedi, H, Forogh, B, Bahramizadeh, M, Keyhani, MR. Effects of insole with toe-separator and night splint on patients with painful hallux valgus: a comparative study. Prosthetics & Orthotics Int. 2008;32(1):79-83

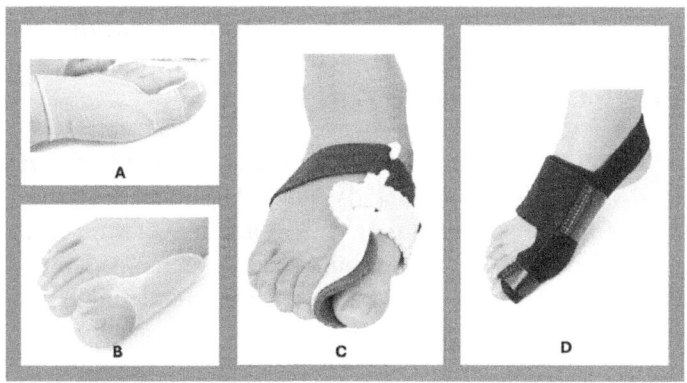

Fig.2.11 A – soft bunion shield (Yogamedic™). B – Avidda bunion sleeve and shield with toe separator. C – Traditional night splint without a tensioner. ZJchao bunion corrector. D – Promifun bunion corrector. The soft splint is valuable after surgical correction once the skin has healed.

Manipulation and night splint

Morne du Plessis published his paper in 2011. This was a joint effort between South Africa, the USA and Australian contributors in *Chiropractic*. Again, a night splint was used as a rigid design. The numbers in the study were the same as Tehraninasar's cohort – thirty divided into two groups. In this case, the difference was the addition of manipulation exercises used in one group with a night splint and the other without.

Du Plessis[31] described the deformity as having *mild to moderate* pain. In this paper, the researchers used the VAS method of assessing pain and a marked questionnaire (Foot Function Index) scheme before and after.

---

[31] Du Plessis, M, Zipfel, B, Brantingham,J, Parkin-Smith, GF, Birdsey, P, Globe, G, Cassa, TK. Manual and manipulative therapy compared to night splint symptomatic hallux abducto-valgus: An exploratory randomised clinical trial. The Foot. 21(2011) 71-78

The score provided a value for improvement. Ideally, the score after treatment is lower than at the start. Additionally, movement was measured.

The follow-up period was a month, and manipulation was added. The night splint and manipulation proved more successful than doing nothing. The authors of this study believed such observations could lead to the consideration of using the manual manipulation technique and night splint before surgery.

Dynamic splint

Christian Plaass[32] published their paper in 2018, the most recent of these three studies. Again, the study focused on symptomatic hallux valgus. Fifty-five patients were used in two study groups: 26 and 29, respectively. The period of follow-up, as with Tehraninasar, was three months. Unlike the other two studies, this was a German team of *orthopaedic surgeons*. The details of the state of the joint were thoroughly documented. Unlike the other studies, a control was added. This meant that twenty-six patients had no treatment during the same period, while twenty-nine were all issued with the designated Halluxsan Splint[TM] [33] (not illustrated – see footnote). As one might expect, the conclusion is that those with the dynamic splint did better than those without treatment. In all cases, there was no change in the angle of deformity, so the joint did not change in position. Pain, however, was minimised and delayed further treatment.

---

[32] Plaass, C, Karch, A, Koch, A, Widederhoeft, V, Ettinger, S, Classen,L, Daniilidis, K, Yao, D, Stukenborg-Colsman, C. Short-term results of dynamic splinting for hallux valgus –A prospective randomized study. Foot and Ankle Surgery 2020; 26 (2):146-150

[33]Halluxsan site shows responsible advertising. https://albrechtgmbh.com/en/produkt/halluxsan/

Kilmartin and MacFarlane provided night splints to 21 children with bunions, for a minimum period of three years. X-rays were taken prior to treatment to measure the degree of the bunion deformity. The children stopped using the splints when their bones stopped growing. A final X-ray was taken at an average of three years after the children stopped using the night splints and the bunion deformity was once again measured on the X-ray.

Over the average seven year period between the start of night splint treatment and the final X-ray measurement there was no deterioration in the bunion deformity. Night splints can therefore prevent the deterioration of bunions in children. In some children the splints did achieve some correction but for most this was not the case[34].

The Clinician's Dilemma

The evidence shows that studies with small recruits make conclusions more difficult than if large study numbers could be recruited. However, small numbers are a reality in orthopaedic work. All studies show that deformity cannot be altered, but symptoms can.

> Taping to the skin cannot be used indefinitely because of damage to the skin. Splints designed along the lines of the Halluxscan make sense as they are adjustable for tension, making them distinctly different from Du Plessis's splint. The splint, or as Plaass describes, "…allows for a prolonged stretch to correct contracted tissue and influence the H.V. (hallux valgus angle) position.

---

[34] MacFarlane AJH, Kilmartin TE. Conservative treatment of juvenile hallux valgus – A seven year prospective study
Br. J. Podiatry 2004; 7:101-105

All patients in the treatment group were instructed to set the adjustable Quengel mechanism, such that there was no perceptible traction, and to wear the brace during their rest time for as long as tolerated."

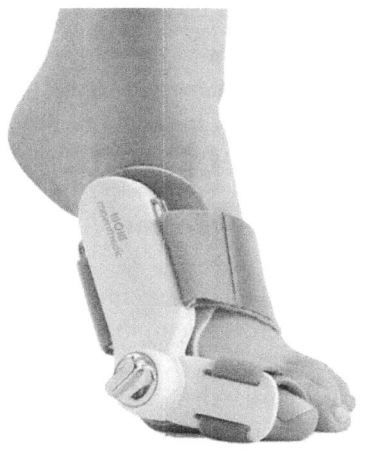

Fig.2.12. An example of a tensioner night splint. It is currently the best type of splint because it is adjustable.

The Quengel mechanism is simply a tensioner mechanism pulling the big toe away from the second toe. Surgery can be averted if patients are willing to try the mechanism but by no means do tensioner splints guarantee that surgery is not inevitable.

One problem with the sales technique and accompanying video is that it suggests the tensioner will increase the correction each day.

While this is possible, the amount of correction of any hallux valgus position will be proportional to the length of time the deformity has been sustained and the extent of the angle of deformity. Using the analogy of the person standing on the edge of a swimming pool, too much lean, and the joint will not recover.

The price of these night splints will vary, but anyone wishing to avoid surgery may benefit from improved comfort. The reapplication is necessary if pain returns, as the benefits from research suggest that relief may only last for a few days!

Non-Surgical Intervention

Who to go to?

If you have exhausted all avenues, from footwear to splints, then seeking assistance is wise. Your next objective should be to obtain a diagnosis and treatment plan. In the UK, patients will probably go to their GP first, in the USA the choice may be wider as many treatment programmes depend on insured cover. In the NHS patients maybe referred to orthopaedic surgeons, although a triage service comprises podiatrists and physiotherapists who prioritise treatment options.

When using the independent (private) sector podiatrists, are the best professionals to seek help, although foot health practitioners and physiotherapists will undoubtedly point you in one direction or another.

A podiatric or orthopaedic surgeon is required for surgical management. Discussion of the merits of one service over another is outside the remit of this book. Websites are one of the ways to seek further information about each person you may wish to seek help from. We can call this next section interactive management to achieve a supportive strategy for progress. There are excellent websites (mentioned earlier) with many clinicians offering video discussion and help sheets.

Compound Bunion Problem

As the hallux valgus increases in size, additional problems arise (Fig.2.14):—

The width of the foot increases. (splayfoot).
Subluxation of the second toe with or without buckling.
Corns over toes, the exostosis bump, in between toes.
Callus under the foot.
Chilblains.
An ever-expanding swelling (cyst) over the exostosis.

The Complete Patient Guide To Bunion Problems.

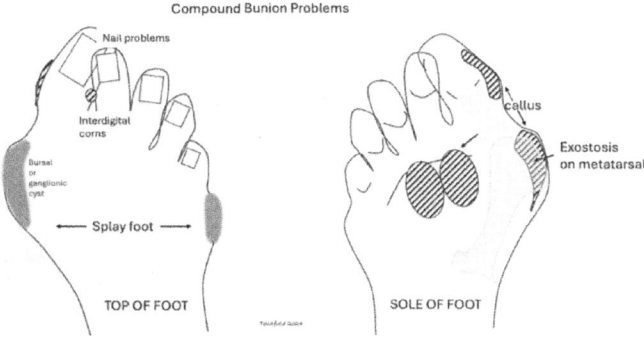

Fig.2.13. Schematic showing common concerns that require professional support. (Tollafield 2024)

The podiatrist's role is to prevent skin damage, maintain mobility, reduce pain and provide foot health education. If you have read the earlier part of the book and understood the range of problems, it becomes more apparent why simple remedies fail over time. Those with 'At Risk' feet from medical disease, poor immunity, and reduced circulation can access NHS podiatry care more readily than those without such problems.

Orthotics (FO)

The foot orthosis (FO) is the preferred name given to a custom insert inside a shoe often prescribed for individual feet to improve foot posture and balance across the forefoot. A foot orthosis (FO) may be designed from heel to toe or run from heel to behind the toes or to the end of the toes. It is not an arch support, but it allows the foot to work by stabilising the forefoot against the hindfoot, influencing muscle balance.

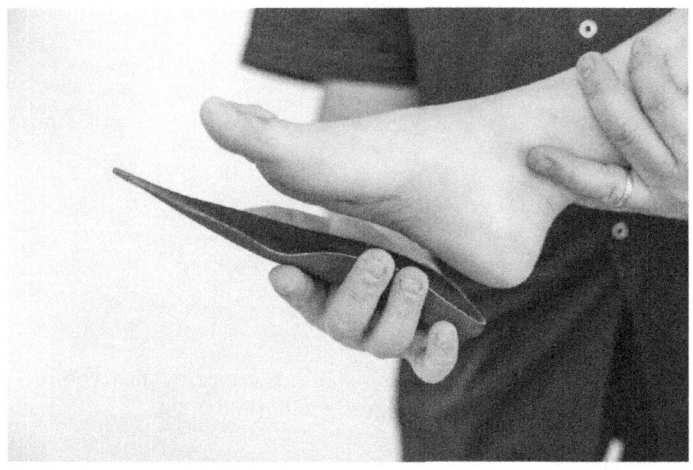

Fig.2.14. A full-length FO fitted after a cast has been taken. This is an example of a bespoke (prescription) device called an inlay or arch support (sic).

More often an orthosis is made of heat-molded thermoplastic or ground out of solid material by computer technology. These differ from insoles as they fit the foot precisely, having been molded from custom casts or different types of impressions rather than sized by the shoe (Fig.2.14). FOs are sold through many outlets, and there is no law in the UK to say who can supply them; many adverts imply unrealistic success, and the opportunity for being misled, high.

The Cochrane database withdrew a nine-year review (Ferrari 2004) because it was outdated, but the paper offers some insight into impartial evidence. The reviewer's conclusion is provided below, and the critique is essential. The dots (ellipses) remove extraneous material, and substituted words are included in brackets.

...few studies had considered conservative treatments. The evidence from these suggested that orthoses and night splints did not appear to be any more beneficial in improving outcomes than no treatment. Surgery ... was shown to be beneficial compared to orthoses or no treatment ... It was notable that the numbers of participants in some trials remaining dissatisfied at follow-up were consistently high (25 to 33%), even when the *hallux valgus* angle and pain had improved [after surgery] ... outcomes were most frequently measured at one year, with a few trials maintaining follow-up for 3 years. ... Future research should include ... longer surveillance periods, more usefully in the region of 5–10 years.

The length of the period of surgical follow-up is more important, and a case study illustrates this point in Part III (surgery). In this second review, the author considers the effect of FOs on the foot with a bunion. Medial pressure refers to the side of the foot alongside the arch.

Significant changes in medial pressure were not seen with the addition of any orthosis compared with standard footwear alone. However, a trend toward increased medial pressures was seen with the full- and sulcus-length [*under the toes*] orthoses, and the 3/4-length orthoses exhibited a trend toward decreased medial pressures. We were unable to demonstrate that the use of a custom foot orthosis significantly decreases the medial pressures on the first metatarsal head in patients with *hallux valgus* deformity. The 3/4-length orthosis was less likely to negatively affect ... pressures, which were noted to increase with ... orthoses.

Our data suggest that if a clinician uses this treatment option, a 3/4-length orthosis might be a better choice than a sulcus or full-length orthosis[35].

There is much debate about the value of orthoses for controlling flexible feet that flatten out; also referred to as pes planus and pronated feet. Many believe flat feet contribute to hallux valgus. However, orthoses are more likely to aid secondary symptoms of metatarsalgia. In some cases, joint pain might diminish as orthoses can reduce movement around the big toe. The use of the FO remains substantially unproven, and yet co-existing foot pain does respond to some FO modalities. Despite modern study methods using force platforms that can measure the loads under the foot, we are unable to develop a standard protocol and confidently say you must have an FO. The patient's choice remains, but it is easy to become trapped with the sales pitch. There is no evidence that HV can be corrected with FO, although some factors can be reduced, such as tendon pain in the flexible flat foot.

Before any surgical correction, conservative treatment should always be initiated first. Currently, there is no consensus that conservative management by shoe modification and foot orthoses could correct the pathology or terminate the clinical worsening of the condition, Colò, G., 2024[36].

---

[35] Doty JF, Harris WT (2018) Hallux valgus deformity and treatment: a three-dimensional approach. Foot Ankle Clin 23(2):271–280. https://doi.org/10.1016/j.fcl.2018.01.007

[36] Colò, G., Leigheb, M., Surace, M.F. *et al.* The efficacy of shoes modification and orthotics in hallux valgus deformity: a comprehensive review of literature. *Musculoskelet Surg* (2024). https://doi.org/10.1007/s12306-024-00839-9

Colò helpfully points out that a three-quarter-length orthosis causes less pressure from shoes, which is increased with full-length orthoses (Fig.2.14). The authors disagree with the study's suggestion that foot orthoses maintain the correct position acquired over time, as the length of time recorded falls short of the period that would reassure patients. However, benefits up to five and even seven years are possible. Few studies appear to correct hallux valgus or reduce its progression (Colò, 2024).

Using expensive custom FOs for hallux valgus are not advised, but secondary or compound problems, including foot fatigue and muscle pain, may benefit. As a rule, allow a size increase to fit an orthosis, especially if the material is thick. Some modern bespoke orthoses are stronger and may require little alteration to footwear. Seek professional advice from a podiatrist.

Aspiration of the Bunion Cyst

If tethering down a ganglion with tape fails and the soft swelling enlarges, the clinician (usually a foot surgeon) will provide a local anaesthetic and draw off fluid using a syringe and needle. This must be done with sterility in mind. Some cysts become loculated, meaning they have several chambers.

The success of aspiration may be temporary, but it serves as an interim method before surgery. The reason for recurrence is that the lining remains and is still easily irritated unless some external factors are corrected or removed. The most typical problem is the underlying exostosis.

> **CASE STUDY – Cyst formation following an arthrodesis**[37]
>
> A 75-year-old had a sizable cyst under her metatarsal, so she was walking on this like a balloon. This was left to develop over 20 years. She had originally had surgery on her big toe, and this was stiffened in an unfortunate position many years earlier. The toe stuck up, and the pressure under her joint was immense, destroying the padding, fat, and surrounding connective tissue, which formed a cyst. There was minimal padding upon surgical removal, although she was given a spongy insole. This case was extreme, but patients do present to the clinic with cysts around the first toe joint, and surgery is necessary. Those diagnosed with severe rheumatoid arthritis formed unpleasant cysts filled with inflammatory cells, causing destruction together with severe dislocation.

Joint Injections

Simple joint inflammation is more common than arthritis and is often referred to as synovitis; an inflamed joint capsule lining. Chronic discomfort may resolve after an injection. Steroids are used in liquid forms mixed with local anaesthetic. Where needle phobia arises, an anaesthetist can use light anaesthesia called sedation.

Needle phobia should never be taken lightly. Single-joint injections are preferred and not advised where there is little benefit. The steroid works by minimising inflammation, and if muscles lying along the sole around the big toe joint have tightened (spasm), the steroid relieves both the pain and the spasm so the joint can move.

---

[37] Arthrodesis is a surgical procedure where a joint is fixed to prevent movement.

If this is the case, then there is a chance this is transient synovitis with spastic muscle contraction, which should settle. Risks from steroid injections are low, but it is possible to have side effects such as a sudden flare-up of pain, which subsides within days. Allergies are rare.

Synovial joint

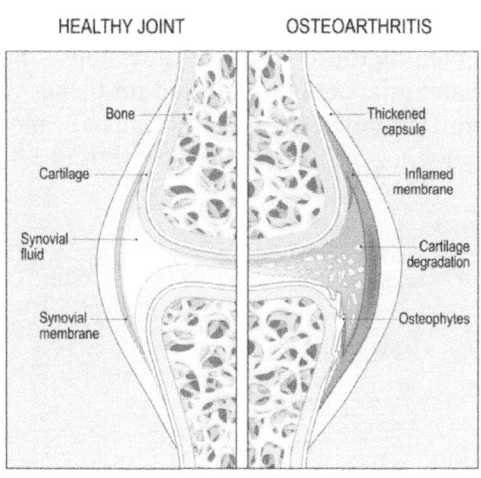

Fig.2.15 Shows a typical synovial joint as in the mtpj. Arthritis (the term arthrosis is also used) is more progressive but can start with inflammation of the synovial lining.

Other toe injections include sodium hyaluronate, a molecular sugar product, but this has yet to enjoy scientific support, and its use appears limited. Hylan G-F 20 was no more effective than a placebo in reducing symptoms in patients with arthrosis (Munteanu 2011).[38]

---

[38] Munteanu, S., Zammit, G.V. & Menz, H.B. Predictors of successful treatment in patients receiving intra-articular injections of hylan G-F 20

Oral forms of glucosamine are marketed but the experience for many people can be disappointing when arthrosis is present. There is no evidence to suggest glucosamine or its supplements will benefit bunion pain.[39]

From clinical experience, using injections for a known deformity such as hallux valgus has limited long-term value.

Injection flares occur in 5-10% of patients and are usually temporary. After that, discomfort reduces, and benefits are more notable. Steroids or other injections, including a dextrose/water mix, are not indicated for hallux valgus as a routine approach unless there is a clear indication of joint damage, synovitis, or muscle spasm.

---

or saline for painful first MTPJ OA. *J Foot Ankle Res* **4** (Suppl 1), P42 (2011). https://doi.org/10.1186/1757-1146-4-S1-P42

[39] Newman, T. 2023. Glucosamine Should I Try It. Medical News Today. On-line Accessed Oct. 2024 Link: https://www.medicalnewstoday.com/articles/265748#what-is-glucosamine

The Complete Patient Guide To Bunion Problems.

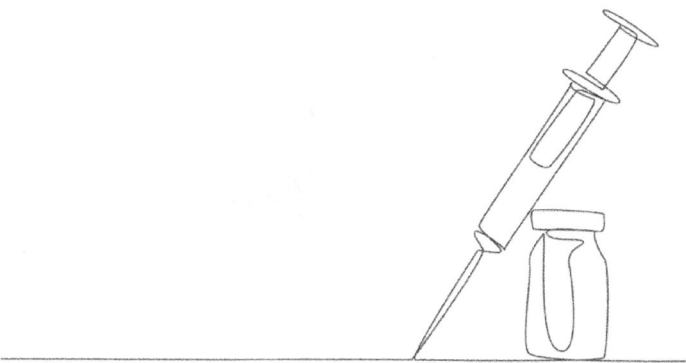

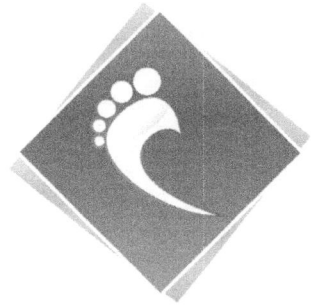

Part II - Summary

Self-help implies ways to manage either the bunion or hallux valgus without clinical intervention. Patients can protect the skin, use splints to assist with pain and rest the part.

Consult a health professional—a podiatrist or foot health practitioner—for further advice if in doubt. It is less expensive than seeking out a surgeon at this stage.

The NHS may be able to offer advice for those in certain categories, but podiatric services have shrunk over the last twenty-five years.

- Try to find a conservative approach to keep you comfortable.
- Surgery in the young is not ideal because bunions can reoccur
- Surgery, later on in life, can be prejudiced by medical problems and depend on bone quality.
- Healing quality diminishes with age.

Who Should I Seek Foot Treatment & Advice From?

General foot problems – Podiatrist or Foot Health practitioners.
Surgery – a podiatric or dedicated orthopaedic foot surgeon

General:

Podiatrists are university-trained and must be registered with the Health and Care Professionals Council (HCPC). NHS and independent practising locations. (3-4 years)

Foot Health Practitioners (FHPs) are self-regulated, and training varies throughout the UK. Podiatry organisations train FHPs and follow similar standards of care up to the level of competency. (12-18 months)

Surgery:

Podiatric surgeons are qualified podiatrists trained in related medicine and surgery dedicated to the foot. They do not deal with trauma but elective, non-emergency surgery. They are registered under the HCPC on a separate register, and newly qualified surgeons must meet current accreditation standards. Podiatric surgeons specialise in daycare surgery. (13 years). A number work within orthopaedic directorates (UK). Royal College of Podiatry—https://rcpod.org.uk/podiatric-surgery/about-podiatric-surgery.

Orthopaedic surgeons are medically qualified doctors registered with the General Medical Council. The number of dedicated foot surgeons has increased over the last thirty years. Orthopaedic surgeons also specialise in trauma. Their training is broader than podiatric surgeons within the medical field. (16 years)—British Orthopaedic Society—https://www.boa.ac.uk/about-us.html.

Both podiatric and orthopaedic surgeons practice in the NHS. *Years given in brackets are approximations only.*

Common Questions

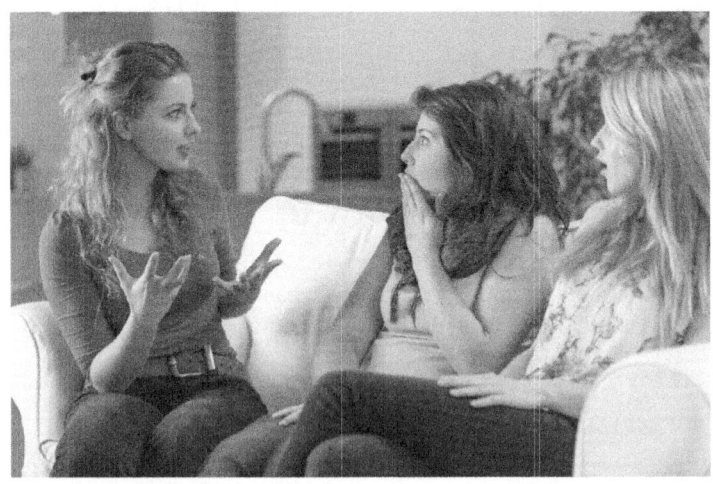

I have a painful bump.

Protect with a silicone or sponge sleeve. Treat infections early using first aid. Always ensure the shoe is designed for your needs and foot size. The broad nature of this question may be the one query you start with. There are some opportunities to help yourself if you are determined, but it is a question of bump (bunion) or deformity (hallux valgus).

If your foot is at risk—poor circulation, lack of nerve sensation, or poor healing—you should be under the care of a professional—podiatrist. Skincare and protection management are critical.

My toe joint painful?

Rest the joint. Use a stiff-soled shoe until the toe settles. Strap the toe for short periods or use a splint. If it hurts when moving and there has been no injury, try an analgesic or even a cold pack if the pain is marked. If there is no improvement by 24-48 hours, seek advice. Taping a toe with fan strapping (see Video -Fig.2.8) can be helpful for short periods and a night splint. Again, after using these techniques for three weeks, seek professional help.

Should I have fluid drained from my foot swelling

It is worth doing if the fluid increases and affects your life. Recurrence arises when the cyst (ganglion or bursa) is well established.

My toe crosses and pushes my second or third toes out of alignment?

Many people try to tape toes together, but this is not a long-term solution and is amenable to surgery. Footwear becomes imperative when selecting size, width and depth. Corn formation and nail problems arise. Seek a professional opinion to guide you.

I have shoe fitting problems?

If you want to fit the wider foot, consider using sites that offer wider shoes. Use an insock to improve the shoe's fit for the smaller, narrower foot. Bespoke or made-to-measure footwear is mainly for at-risk patients. Bootees and central top open zip shoes are helpful for older patients or where pressure must be minimised. Where shoe fit ultimately impacts footwear, bunion surgery will make a difference by narrowing the foot and changing your shoe size.

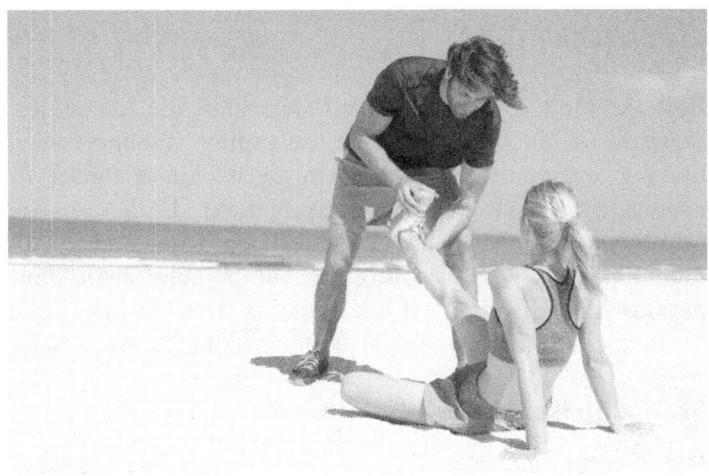

My foot is unsightly—I hate going to the beach.

While we do not advocate surgery for cosmetic reasons, we understand how the psychology of appearance can affect patients. Remember, many people have bunions, including those in the Hall of Fame. Do not be ashamed, as many people have this shape. If it does not hurt, try to accept your foot's appearance. If all fails, consult a surgeon, but remember that you may be worse off, which can be as much as 2-5%.

I don't want my foot to become worse.

Many do not want feet like an older relative. First, consider your family and whether those who suffered had treatment. Did the hallux valgus worsen? If not, accept the problem, size your feet to fit the shoe, and make the correct selection. This alone is not an ideal reason to have surgery, and the risks must again be appreciated. Parts III and IV will deal with many of these concerns. However, find out as much information about your relative as possible and seek an opinion from a surgeon. If, on the other hand, the foot does deteriorate with pain and compound problems, then surgery may be an option for you.

I am plagued with corn and hard skin.

Seek assistance and a treatment plan from a podiatrist. You can manage simple callus with creams and safe abrasive modalities. Skin thickening occurs due to overuse, blister formation, incorrect footwear for the job at hand, and bone and joint deformity. Manage light thickening with regular softening creams after bathing. Avoid corn plasters over joints—these can cause ulcers and infection. Reduce skin with safety in mind, including using rotary sanders designed for the job (not the DIY type of sander!).

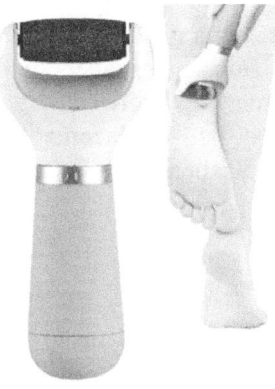

Fig.2.16 Rotary sander for callus

We suggest avoiding sharp instruments, but alternatives, as shown, include chiropody sponges, pumice stones, and the sander system. There are always contra-indications, such as poor circulation, fragile skin, numb skin and sensation (neuropathy). While the foot does not suffer from many malignant conditions, be careful with blemishes that appear and seek a medical opinion before attempting to remove skin around the site.

Part III

This section is reserved for those seeking foot surgery. While podiatrists in the UK can offer advice, you will find more than enough information in this book to lead you to the next stage—the surgical consultation.

With so many surgical options, we need to ensure that readers understand the difference between osteotomies, arthrodesis, replacement joints and arthroplasties versus osteotomies.

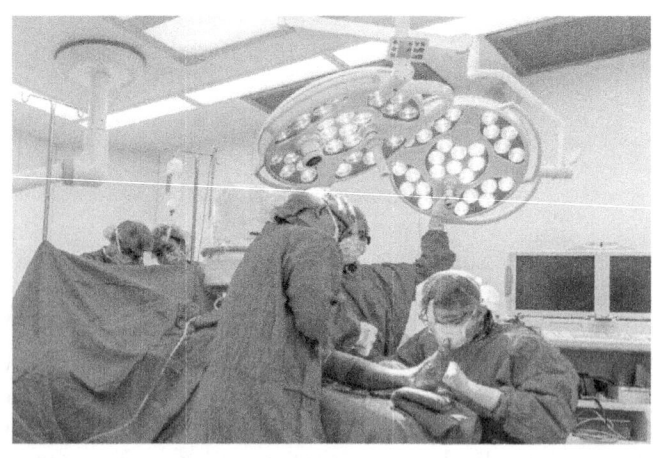

Foot Surgery for Bunions

Making the Decision

If you were me, what would you do?—This is a question often asked by patients suffering from problems associated with their bunion. We know only too well that some would like the surgeon to make the decision for them, but that would be poor practice. Patients need to be involved in the decision; our role is to guide them to make the right decision for them as individuals.

Follow your instincts —You will know when you can't live with the problem any longer.

How much of a problem is it?—If the bunion is causing regular and significant pain and is restricting your lifestyle, then surgery has a lot to offer. If you can manage the situation easily, footwear is not too much of an issue, you can do all the things you want to do without restriction and you are rarely in significant pain then there is certainly no need to rush into surgery.

There are three reasons for undergoing bunion surgery:—

- First and foremost, pain.
- Secondly, if you cannot find any shoes to fit, that will drive a lot of people into undergoing surgery.
- Thirdly, if the bunion is now beginning to involve the second toe, causing it to be pushed upwards and backwards into a hammer toe, or it is beginning to cross over the big toe, or you are feeling like you are walking on marbles on the ball of your foot then surgery is strongly indicated.

At this point the problem is no longer just an issue of the big toe joint but is progressively involving the whole foot. Most patients who opt for surgery present all three reasons, though the severity of their problems will vary markedly. Like everything, bunions can be mild, moderate, or severe, and the pain associated with the problem can be likewise. As a rule of thumb, if pain is 6/10 or more on a visual analogue scale, then the patient's pain is sufficient to warrant surgery.

PAIN MEASUREMENT SCALE

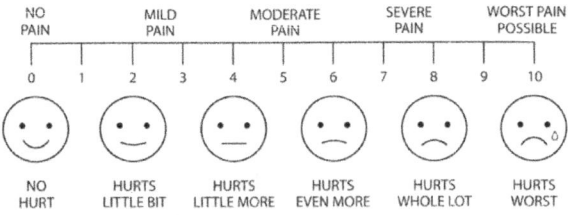

Fig.3.1. Visual analogue scales are designed to assist patients in determining how a problem impacts on their tolerance of discomfort.

Is pain the best reason for undergoing surgery?

This can be problematic; it is not uncommon for young patients to present with mild bunions but with significant pain, which is disproportionate to the severity of the bunion. In such cases, it is essential that non-surgical treatments like in-shoe orthotics and cortisone injections are tried in the first instance, as it is possible that surgery can be avoided. On the other end of the spectrum, it is common for bunion sufferers to present with very marked bunion deformity but with little or no pain. This is usually because they are managing the situation with careful footwear selection. In those cases, surgery is still indicated if there are significant problems with shoe fitting or the bunion is deforming the other toes. Pain is an important consideration but not the only reason for undergoing surgery.

> In cases of mild deformity but a lot of pain, surely it is best to undergo surgery sooner rather than later as it will only get worse.

It is not uncommon for experienced clinicians to see patients in their late teens to thirties who present with very mild deformity but severe pain, which they will often rate as 8 to 10 on a visual analogue scale. This is referred to as disproportionate pain, and it can often prove very unpredictable in its response to surgical correction of the bunion.

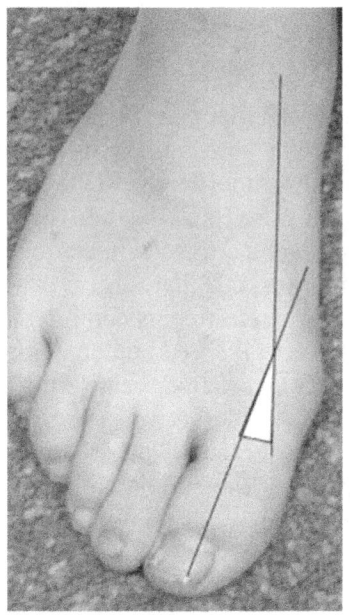

Fig.3.2. Mild deformity and a low angle is shown.
(Tollafield 2016)

Of particular concern is that surgical correction of a mild hallux valgus can, in our experience, frequently result in stiffness of the big toe joint, which will also be associated with pain and restriction of activities and footwear choice.

In one study[40] which looked at the outcome of bunion surgery in fifty women who had undergone bunion surgery nine years previously, there was an 8% incidence of painful stiffness of the big toe joint following surgery.

---

[40] Kilmartin TE O'Kane C. Combined rotation scarf Akin osteotomies for hallux valgus; a patient focused 9 year follow up of 50 patients J. Foot Ankle Research 2010, 3:2. Available at http://www.jfootankleres.com/content/3/1/2)

This is a significant complication, patients are rarely happy with their surgical result if the big toe joint is stiff. Stiffness will cause pain as the joint will jam with every step. It will also impact the style of walking, with sufferers being forced to take smaller steps and change their footwear as there is simply not enough upward movement of the toe to allow higher heels to be worn as the position of the big toe joint in high heels demands more upward movement of the big toe.

Nine Year Follow-up

In that same study, which looked at women nine years after their surgery, 14% were unable to wear high-heeled shoes nine years after their operation.

Surgical treatment is to be avoided in mild deformities without pain because of the risk of stiffness. Often, the pain of the condition can be alleviated with cortisone injections, which are very powerful anti-inflammatory drugs. These injections switch off inflammation in the big toe joint, which then resolves the pain.

> Why does stiffness occur in mild bunion deformities?

In severe bunions, the soft tissue sleeve, known as the joint capsule, is stretched and thinned by the malalignment of the big toe. In mild deformities, the capsule is not as flexible, so when it is divided at surgery to allow access to the underlying bone, it scars and tightens, which then manifests as joint stiffness.

The importance of the movement of the big toe joint

The big toe's upward movement is necessary to allow you to push off from the ground. In the normal foot, there should be a minimum of 40° of upward movement. If the toe's upward movement is limited, it will also restrict activities like crouching, lunging, or standing on tip toes.

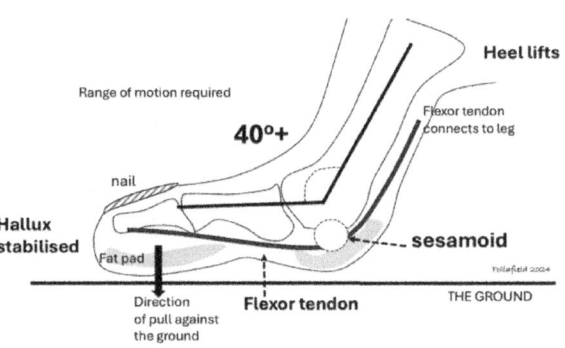

Fig.3.3 Push-off requires a stable to on the ground associated with downward movement.

Downward movement of the big toe is also important for pushing off the ground. If there is restricted movement or reduced downward power/strength in the big toe it will no longer feel so natural to push off from the ground with every step. Worse still it can lead to a subconscious guarding of the foot which means that you push off from the smaller toes rather than the big toe. By throwing your weight away from the big toe it then overloads the smaller joints on the ball of the foot which in time become bruised and then inflamed.

This is a condition known as transfer metatarsalgia and can be caused by bunions or can also develop after bunion surgery. In those cases where metatarsalgia is a complication of bunion surgery and the risk of it developing it should have been discussed before the operation as part of the informed consent process.

Informed Consent For Surgery

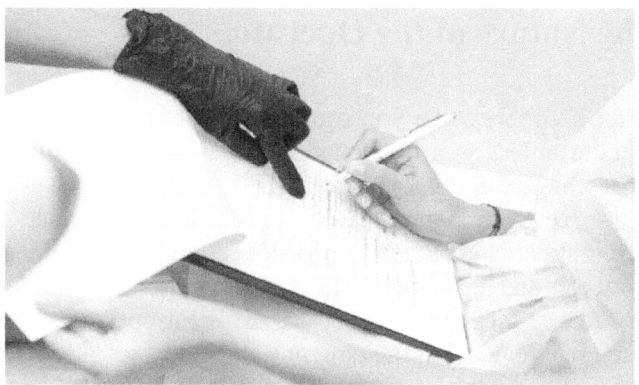

By the time in life that you need an operation to correct a bunion deformity, you may well have signed many consent forms for other procedures.

Signing the consent form is just one part of the whole process of informed consent. It starts with the discussion of whether you need to have an operation or would it be better to try other non-surgical treatments or even leave well alone. Avoiding any treatment is often the best advice if there is no pain, no footwear fitting difficulties and only minimal deformity which has not involved the other toes.

If both patient and surgeon agree that surgery would be more appropriate than other treatment, the surgeon will discuss the following:—

- The nature of the operation.
- The recovery time and what impact that will have on lifestyle and ability to work.
- The risks and complications of surgery.

The Nature of the Operation

In the same way that you should never invest in a financial scheme unless you understand it, you need to understand what you are letting yourself in for with bunion surgery. There are a number of different procedures with markedly different demands in terms of recovery and return to normal footwear and activities. The fact that there are different procedures means that there are different options and best practice dictates that the patient will be advised about those options and then the advice will focus on what the surgeon considers as the best option for the individual.

Understanding the recovery time is critical to achieve a good outcome. It takes approximately fourteen days for the outside of a wound to heal following surgery to the foot. In that time it is vital that the foot is rested as too much activity will cause significant swelling as the body struggles to heal the foot after the trauma of the operation.

Too much walking and standing in the first two weeks after surgery can make the foot sufficiently swollen that the wound may open up slightly delaying recovery. Following most bunion operations, the optimum time off work is six weeks. Swelling remains an important limiting factor.

Nowhere in the whole body swells as much as the foot does after surgery and nowhere stays so swollen for so long. The reason for this is gravity. Gravity pulls blood and tissue fluid down into the foot and keeps it there. Blood and fluid are vital to repair the surgery site, but it will also give rise to a range of symptoms, including pins and needles, aching, burning, tightening, stretching, tearing and heaviness.

As time passes, the swelling improves but takes six weeks to improve to the point when return to work is possible, and three to five months before it has resolved completely.

If you do not have six weeks to rest and take things slowly, your recovery will be delayed, and the swelling may become more protracted.

Risks & Complications of Surgery

Complications of bunion surgery can be minor to severe, fleeting or permanent, as well as life-changing. Whilst most complications are nothing more than a temporary setback on the road to recovery, some can have a serious impact on your future lifestyle. Because complications are a fact of any surgical intervention, most surgeons will be reluctant to operate on a condition that is mild and causing minimal pain or inconvenience. Simply put, the stakes are high in such a situation because even if a minor complication develops following surgery, it will be the case that the patient is now worse off than they were before surgery.

So what can go wrong? The following paragraphs will consider the types of complications and their significance in terms of impact on the patient's life and lifestyle. To further explain the importance of the complication, the incidence of these problems will be presented. This is based upon a study which followed fifty female patients up to nine years after their bunion surgery.

Further evidence of the incidence of complications is taken from the Faculty of Podiatric Surgery National Audit of Podiatric Surgeons (PASCOM-10)[41].

Stiffness of the big toe joint following bunion surgery. There is a 3% risk. The impact on lifestyle is moderately high.

If the big toe joint is stiff following surgery, it is doubtful that the patient will be happy. As described earlier, stiffness is often associated with pain but also significant footwear and activity restrictions. In many cases, the problem can improve and eventually resolve up to a year following surgery, but some don't, and further treatment is required, including cortisone injections and manipulation under anaesthetic to try and force more movement into the big toe joint.

Pressure transfer to the ball of the foot. 2% risk. Impact on lifestyle: moderately high.

This condition, called transfer metatarsalgia, Fig.3.4, causes a sensation of walking on marbles on the ball of the foot. It is a consequence of weakness or shortening of the big toe bones. It limits walking distance and footwear choice because in order to alleviate it, thick-soled shoes like trainers need to be worn. The problem can be relieved by restoring strength to the big toe or using insoles that cushion and offload the pressure on the 2nd and 3rd metatarsophalangeal joints. If this fails, further surgery may

---

[41] PASCOM-10 was originally developed in 1997 and adopted by the now Royal College of Podiatry. From 2010 the system was developed to encompass training of podiatric surgeons. https://www.pascom-10.com

be necessary.

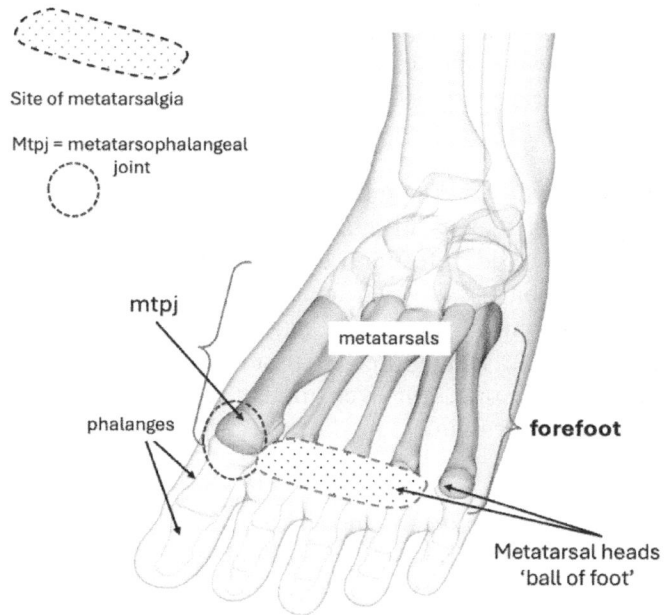

Site of metatarsalgia

Mtpj = metatarsophalangeal joint

mtpj

metatarsals

phalanges

forefoot

Metatarsal heads 'ball of foot'

Fig.3.4 Site of transfer metatarsalgia.

Overcorrection. 4% risk. Impact on lifestyle: high.

If the big toe is made too straight by surgery, it gives rise to a range of symptoms, including stiffness of the big toe joint, pain on the ball of the foot, and shoe-fitting problems, as the big toe cannot easily be accommodated in a normal toe box. Further surgery to reduce the overcorrection is usually necessary.

> Infection or wound healing problems 2% risk. Impact on lifestyle: Usually mild and short term, but if infection is severe, the impact can be limb and life threatening.

Infection destroys skin and the tissues underlying the skin, causing pain that is difficult to control even with strong painkillers. Mild infections can usually be cleared with antibiotic tablets, but when severe, especially if it involves bone, intravenous antibiotics may be required and even surgery to cut away infected tissue. Fortunately, severe infections are rare, but even mild infections will always delay wound healing.

> Deep vein thrombosis Less than 1% risk. Impact on lifestyle: high.

Immobilisation is inevitable following foot surgery. With immobilisation, the muscles of the leg are no longer so active, and this leads to reduced function of the so-called calf muscle pump, which is a way of describing how the big muscles of the calf squeeze the blood in the deep veins of the leg back in the direction of the heart.

When the activity of the calf muscle pump reduces as the patient is forced to rest, the blood may pool and then form a blood clot, which blocks the vein. The blood clot is then at risk of eventually dislodging and moving into the general circulation, where it may block the lungs, forming a pulmonary embolism or a pressure blockage in the brain, which can kill brain tissue, manifesting as a stroke.

Pain syndrome. Less than 1% risk.
Impact on lifestyle: Very high.

In the hours and days following a bunion operation, some level of pain is inevitable. In order to minimise pain a combination of local anaesthetic nerve blocks, at the time of your surgery, and painkillers provided after your surgery will make an impact on reducing discomfort. Advice on how to rest, elevate and ice the foot to minimise swelling, will also alleviate help to alleviate pain.

Pain will most likely subside after three to four days, and the need for regular painkillers diminishes. However, for some patients, this normal pathway does not happen. Pain proves difficult to control from the start, and as the days pass, it does not diminish but intensifies. In those cases, there is always a concern that they may be developing a complication called complex regional pain syndrome. One way of explaining this rare but catastrophic complication is that following the bunion operation, the trauma of the surgery will inevitably turn on the pain tap. After three or four days, that pain tap should turn off automatically as the body repairs the surgical site. In the pain syndrome condition, the pain tap does not turn off; if anything, the flow increases. Intense, unresolvable pain will lead to myriad consequences, including restricted ability to use the foot, wasting of the muscles of the leg and foot, temperature changes with the foot alternating from feeling ice cold to burning hot, but all the time, there may be increased sweating. Inevitably, chronic pain will give rise to sleeplessness, depression and anxiety.

Complex regional pain syndrome may develop after any form of injury to the body and is best treated by a multidisciplinary team, including pain specialists, physiotherapists, and psychologists, who can help with strategies to manage the pain.

Need to remove metalwork which has been used to fix the bones together. 1.5% risk with certain operations. Impact on lifestyle: low.

Screws, metal bars (plates), and wires fix bones into the correct position and are now standard for almost all bunion operations.

Originally developed by Swiss Surgeons to fix broken bones in Alpine skiers, fixation devices have massively improved recovery time allowing earlier mobility. However, there is one important disadvantage: sometimes, the fixation devices can irritate the soft tissues that overlie the bone. For the patient, this will most commonly manifest as a feeling of a hard lump under the skin irritated by shoes. Sometimes the screw or wire backs out of the bone and breaks the skin surface.

Loosening arises within the bone because the physical properties of the metal is different from the physical properties of bone. Over time the two can begin to repel each other like magnets. On weightbearing, bone flexes and bends, not by huge amounts, in fact it is referred to as micromovement but this movement over long periods is enough to 'work' the screw or the wire out of the bone.

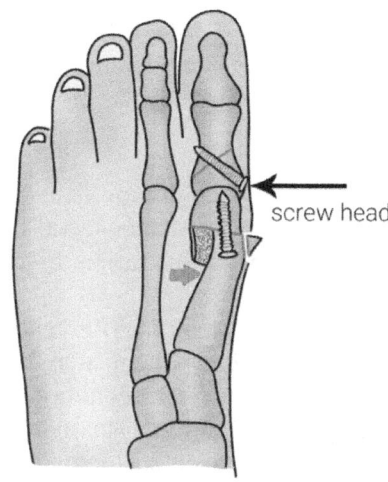

screw head

Fig.3.5 Two screws shown fix the bone for osteotomy surgery. Although a low risk of 1.5%, constant irritation may necessitate removal.

If the fixation screw becomes a source of irritation it is easily resolved by removal. Patients worry when this is proposed to them because it is assumed that screw fixation is still required to hold the bones together, but in fact, as long as the bone has healed, they are quite superfluous after about six weeks. Fixation devices (pins, screws and plates) are constantly evolving in a quest to, among other innovations, make them as low profile as possible and, therefore, ensure they are less likely to irritate the soft tissues overlying the bone.

Fracture of the bone that has been operated on. Up to 1.25% risk. Impact on lifestyle: moderate but usually temporary, occasionally prolonged.

Surgical correction of the bunion deformity does, in many operations, require the first metatarsal bone to be cut, re-aligned and then fixed with fixation. Fig.3.5.

Cutting the bone (osteotomy) inevitably weakens the structure and leaves the patient at risk of fracture either during the operation or, more commonly, in the first days and weeks after the operation. Usually, the fracture is easily detected using X-rays taken postoperatively.

In many cases, it may be dealt with by immobilising the foot in a plastic cast or in special walking boot which has inflatable air cells inside the boot to secure and immobilise the foot (Fig.4.4). Where a fracture is unstable, further surgery may be required. In both scenarios, the foot will be immobilised in the cast or boot for up to six weeks.

Altered Mechanics

The significance of secondary breaks in bone can lead to the first metatarsal being shortened by a fracture, or if the fracture is unstable, it may lead to displacement of the bone upwards, relative to the floor. This can profoundly affect the weight distribution on the ball of the foot and give rise to the metatarsalgia or pain on the ball of the foot described earlier.

Types of Hallux Valgus Surgery

It is helpful to consider three levels that make up a simple classification: minor, intermediate and severe (Fig. 3.5).

Surgery will usually address the shape of the bone and straighten the metatarsal or may include the toe bone (phalanx) so that two bone cuts are made. A cut in bone is called an 'osteotomy,' and joint removal (excision) is called an 'arthroplasty.' For completeness, we have also added the other term, arthrodesis or stiffening. The osteotomy often moves bone in one or more directions to improve function around the joint.

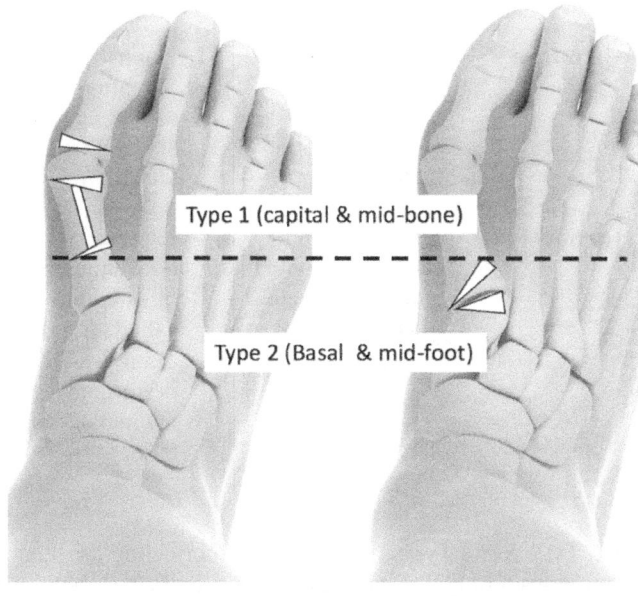

Fig.3.5. Type 1 and Type 2 osteotomy cuts. Bone cuts are positioned depending on the severity of the deformity. The cuts shown are diagrammatic and not intended to be accurate.

	Type 1	**Type 2**
Osteotomy	Chevron (Austin) – metatarsal head. Scarf – metatarsal shaft. Youngswick – metatarsal head. Reverdin Green – metatarsal head. Akin (combined with the others as required) – phalanx.	Basal or basilar osteotomy – metatarsal base.
Arthroplasty	Keller excisional arthroplasty. Replacement (Swanson*) arthroplasty.	Not a primary operation, except in specific cases (see text).
Arthrodesis	Minimal joint surface removal is often associated with stiffening (arthrodesis).	Lapidus (stiffening type of osteotomy is called an arthrodesis) performed at the metatarsal base.

Table 1. Type 1 and Type 2 approaches to correcting the bunion: Bone surgeries will be referred to as Type 1 or Type 2, but this is used merely to distinguish the two different parts of the foot the surgery. *Note: Swanson was the name of the first commercially viable implant that is still used today.

Type 1 uses the middle (shaft) or head (capital) of the bone. Type 2, being rarer in frequency, target larger deformities.

The more common forms used have been named. Not all options are included, and surgeons will have different preferences.

Minimal Incision or Keyhole Bunion Surgery

Minimal incision surgery (MIS), sometimes referred to as keyhole surgery, is far from new and was first described in the 1940s. The MIS surgeon will usually work through three small incisions placed at the side of the big toe joint. The thickening at the side of the mtpj and the bones on either side of the joint are then cut through with a burr.

Temporary wires are used to toggle the bones into a corrected position before screws are introduced to fix the bones in the corrected position. The screws are buried deep in the bone. The whole operation is performed using X-rays at intervals to establish where and how the bones are cut and then how much correction is achieved. After surgery a dressing or cast may be applied to support the foot until the bones heal.

Over the last ten years, extensive research has investigated the effectiveness, safety and patient satisfaction with keyhole surgery techniques. On almost every level, the results of keyhole surgery have been found to be similar to those of open surgery techniques.

In 2024 a comprehensive review of all the keyhole bunion research was performed by the National Institute for Health and Care Excellence (NICE)[42] who found that when open surgery was compared directly with keyhole surgery, the differences were that patients had slightly less pain immediately postoperatively in keyhole surgery. Irritation from the screws used to fix the bones was marginally higher in the keyhole surgery group. Radiation exposure in the keyhole group was fourteen times higher.

One question that remains unanswered is whether keyhole surgery allows a quicker return to normal footwear and activities when the two surgical approaches are compared. On reviewing all the other outcomes, it is likely that this factor will again be similar when keyhole and open surgery are compared.

Whilst it is very likely that keyhole bunion surgery will become increasingly available, it is a very demanding surgical technique, and like all bunion surgery, the best results will be achieved by those surgeons who do it well. Foot surgeons who are already achieving excellent results in open surgery are not necessarily going to rush to develop another technique with potentially disappointing results for their patients. It is possible that further research will find that the greatest advantage of the keyhole techniques is that the smaller incisions reduce the risk of wound healing problems and consequent infection. They could therefore be particularly useful for people with higher surgical infection risk such as diabetics or other health problems which can delay wound healing. More research on these types of patient is awaited.

---

[42] IP 782/2 [IPG789] IP overview: Minimal invasive percutaneous surgical techniques with internal fixation for correcting hallux valgus © NICE 2024.

Preparing For Surgery

Bunion surgery, like all surgery, is deeply inconvenient and very disruptive of everyday day-to-day life. That may sound obvious, but it is surprising how often this can be overlooked by surgery patients. A great deal of personal organisation, from how you are transported to and from the hospital to what you will eat and how you will prepare it, is vital to ensure the best possible recovery.

A key question for all bunion surgery patients is how you can minimise weight-bearing while maintaining enough mobility to reduce the risk of deep vein thrombosis.

Pre-operative rehabilitation in bunion surgery plays a role in recovery. The most important muscles of the big toe joint are the flexor muscles which allow you to grasp the big toe downwards. To illustrate this, these are the muscles that you would need to use if you were to pick a pencil off the floor with your big toe. The stronger these muscles are pre-operatively, the stronger they will be post-operatively. With strong, big-toe (hallux) flexor muscles, it is possible to maintain normal weight distribution much more readily on the ball of the foot.

Weakness of the flexor muscles reduces big toe function and automatically leads to a transfer of weight to the second toe metatarsal bone on the ball of the foot (Fig.3.4) which will feel like walking on a marble. The exercises used to strengthen the flexor muscles will also help reduce the risk of stiffness post operatively. The greater the range of motion pre-operatively, the more likely it is to be maintained post-operatively. There are some reversible reasons for marked pre-operative stiffness of the big toe joint, but these must be identified by the surgeon because they will significantly affect the likely outcome of surgery and therefore should be addressed as part of the operation.

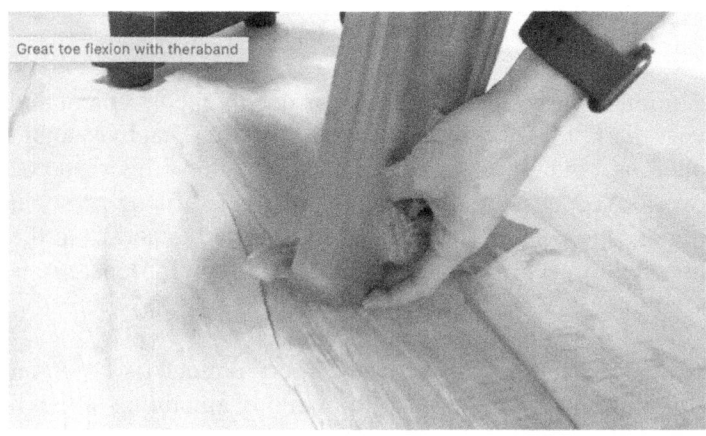

Fig. 3.7. Pre-operative strengthening muscles

Flexor power exercises are simple to perform, they can be done at any time and in terms of equipment all that is required is a powerband. The video from YouTube[43] is helpful—'Great Toe Flexion with Theraband'.

The powerband is basically a big elastic band which allows the hallux to be flexed against the resistance of the elastic band. As the power of the big toe flexor muscle increases the number of repetitions and indeed the amount of stretch or resistance put on the band can be increased.

The best way of performing the flexor power exercises is to sit on a couch with the knee slightly bent and the heel on the couch. Loop the powerband around the big toe and then begin flexing the big toe downwards. Start with the band on light stretch and do this five times.

---

[43] Theraband exercise for toe.
https://video.search.yahoo.com/search/video?fr=aaplw&ei=utf-8&p=theraband+exercises+for+big+toe+joint#action=view&id=1&vid=89bd4ac96ca40ab132b6383cb45b6caf

Then pull the band to medium stretch and flex the big toe three times, then pull the band to full stretch and flex the big toe twice. Repeat this at least three times but preferably five times daily.

Immediately after surgery, it can be difficult to perform this flexor power exercise because of swelling around the big toe joint which restricts movement of the joint. Nevertheless even if the big toe is moving only slightly at first, the movement and strength will continue to improve with repeated exercises.

Nutrition & Vitamin Deficiencies

Malnourished patients are not good candidates for bunion surgery because wound healing can be slowed; this leaves the patient at a higher risk of infection of the wound as the longer the wound remains unhealed, the higher the infection risk.

There may be some benefit in taking vitamin C and D supplements before surgery. Certainly, before considering operations involving fusing the joints of the big toe, it may be helpful to have a blood test to establish that vitamin D levels are normal if your clinician feels a need. If reduced, the patient is asked to take a daily oral dose of between 800 and 20,000 units of cholecalciferol vitamin D for 14 days before surgery. Low vitamin D levels leave the patient at risk of poor bone healing, which, in the case of fusion operations, will almost certainly require further surgery.

Hospital Admission

NHS and hospitals in the independent (private) sector will admit patients either first thing in the morning between 7.30 -8.00 hrs or 12.00 - 13.00 hrs for the afternoon theatre session. Private hospitals will also admit patients around 4.30 pm for evening theatre sessions. Much will depend on whether the planned operation is due to be performed under general anaesthetic, sedation and local anaesthetic or just local anaesthetic.

If you are fully awake and under local anaesthetic, you are likely to spend the shortest time in the hospital. If a general anaesthetic or sedation is used, you will be in the hospital for longer depending upon the speed of your recovery and ability to pass water afterwards.

An anaesthetist will perform a pre-operative assessment at the start of the session, visiting each patient before the theatre session begins. Encountering any wait before being called to the operating theatre makes one anxious.

Whether you are first or last on the list of patients to be operated on will be determined by equipment requirements, the likely duration of your operation and the types of procedures that the other patients on the list are undergoing.

The order of the list is carefully considered by hospital staff to ensure the session runs efficiently so be prepared to wait. Bring something to entertain yourself with. There is nothing to be gained by complaining about your place on the list other than disrupting the theatre session as the surgeon will have to leave theatre to explain why the list has been configured in the way it has.

If undergoing general anaesthetic or sedation, you will need to fast for at least 8 hours prior to surgery. The reason for this is to reduce the risk of vomiting which can be inhaled into the lungs and cause pneumonia.

Upon admission, your identity will be checked on numerous occasions. This is done in conjunction with checking your consent form and is part of a strict hospital procedure to ensure that the correct operation is done on the right body part. It may be tedious to repeatedly be asked for your name and date of birth, but the patient plays a vital role in ensuring the correct procedure is performed to avoid mistakes. The foot is marked with a felt pen skin marker to ensure the correct site is treated. Never feel embarrassed to question any incorrect mark.

If a nerve block is to be performed on the leg and/or ankle, that will also have to be marked with a skin marker.

Wear loose-fitting and easily removed shoes and clothes to your surgery appointment. You will be asked to remove some or all your clothes and change into a theatre gown. This is to ensure you enter the operating theatre in clean garments but also allows easier access for blood pressure monitoring, nerve block and placement of the tourniquet. Remove all nail varnish before surgery—this minimises the risk of flakes of nail varnish penetrating the wound but also helps monitor the circulating blood supply to the toe. The circulation to your fingers will also be monitored during the operation using a pulse oximeter which determines the oxygen levels in your blood. This will not work if the fingernails are varnished.

In Part IV, patients write about their admission experience. In this section, we describe the process from the clinician's point of view and so it is not necessary to watch these unless you want to understand the clinical protocols.

The videos are a few years old but many of the principles of practice remain.

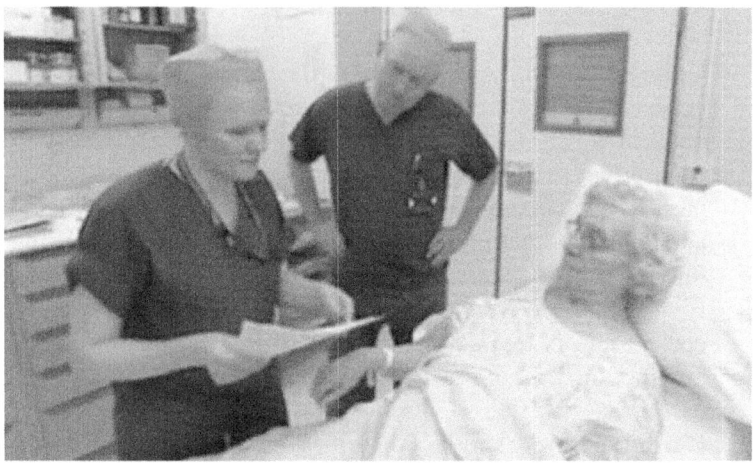

Fig.3.8. The Anaesthetic Room

The National Health Service provides a helpful <u>video</u> on admission to theatre[44], produced by the National Patient Safety Agency (2009).

The University Hospitals Bristol has also produced short videos on admission. (2021), and for <u>Undergoing day-case surgery</u> at University Hospitals Bristol (2018)[45]. The summary in the table below is taken from the author's (DRT) personal experience in 2023 as a patient in the independent sector[46]. The system follows similar protocols to the NHS.

---

[44] The link is https://www.youtube.com/watch?v=CsNpfMldtyk
[45] https://www.youtube.com/watch?v=gB4M9LYqDiE
[46] Tollafield DR. <u>Shoulder Pain-The rotator Cuff Repair.</u> My Journey-Clinician Turned Patient. 2024 Busypencilcase Communications. P:56-7

The Complete Patient Guide To Bunion Problems.

SUMMARY OF ADMISSION

Reception admission (I already had a pre-op check 2 weeks beforehand).

Collection to the room from reception & initial nurse introduction and outline.

Physiotherapy visit and advice about what to expect regarding recovery.

At some point the catering staff take your post-surgery meal order. You can only drink water up to a few hours before but no food from midnight before the day of surgery.

A pharmacist checked and discussed pain control and any other medications I was taking. Hospitals prefer you to leave medicines at home, so you don't accidentally overdose or mix prescriptions.

The anaesthetist visited and conducted verbal consent. This assures fitness to proceed (for him, not you). There are risks with anaesthetics but are notably low. Damage to the nerve is something mentioned which can lead to weakness or permanent changes, but again is low because the anaesthetist uses ultrasound imaging to guide the needle accurately.

The surgeon visited to undertake the consent and mark the shoulder to be operated. You agree to the location of the operation.

Anaesthetic Options

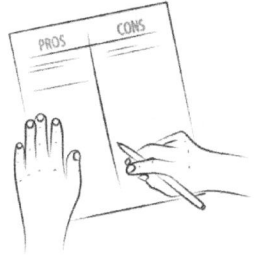

This is an important consideration for any non-emergency operation. You have a choice to undergo your bunion operation whilst fully awake but under local anaesthetic.

Alternatively, you may want to be fully asleep under general anaesthetic or, the last option, something of a halfway house between awake and sleeping where you are under a combination of sedation and local anaesthetic.

Not everywhere can offer all options; some clinics/hospitals may only offer you full general anaesthetic, whereas others only have facilities for local anaesthetic.

Local Anaesthetic

Local anaesthetic offers a much quicker hospital experience. It is likely that the local anaesthetic injections will commence very soon after you are admitted because it can take 45 minutes or more for them to take effect. For bunion surgery, an ankle block is the usual form of local anaesthetic, which involves several injections around your ankle.

For each injection you will feel a sharp scratch and then some pressure under the skin. Most patients consider the discomfort to be mild. Sometimes, however, the injection can come close to the nerve, which is very uncomfortable, but the clinician will quickly adjust the position to stop the discomfort.

Various methods, such as ultrasound and nerve stimulators, are used today to make local anaesthetics safer and more accurate.

The stimulator causes twitching of the foot as the needle moves close to the nerve, affording accuracy.

An anaesthetic block provided behind the knee (popliteal block), provides complete numbness and loss of muscle power in the foot for periods of up to 20 hours. The first night after the operation benefits sleep if pain can be eradicated.

Spinal anaesthetic

Spinal anaesthesia is another form of local anaesthetic. An anaesthetist injects a relatively small volume of local anaesthetic around the spinal cord, making both legs entirely numb. The numbness also affects the bladder, so an essential part of monitoring after surgery includes being able to pass urine before being discharged from care.

An anaesthetist is a specially trained medical doctor who administers general anaesthetic and sedation. Prior to undergoing general anaesthetic or sedation, the anaesthetist must be aware of all your medication and past medical history, as this can have implications for how you react to the drugs administered during general anaesthetic. Similar drugs are used for sedation, but the amounts administered are less, so the patient is not taken to the same level of unconsciousness. Nevertheless, with sedation, the patient is likely to be unaware of their surroundings or even discomfort-producing procedures like local anaesthetic injections.

General Anaesthetic

General anaesthetic can take longer to fully recover, but the difference is that recovery from sedation is usually shorter. The best advice for any patient is that they follow their instincts and if they are perfectly at ease with the idea of being fully awake during their operation, they should opt for local anaesthetic, but if they are very anxious about the whole procedure, it is kinder to receive a general anaesthetic or sedation. Modern surgery today should not invoke unnecessary anxiety as this can be managed to avoid patient concerns.

Recovery After Surgery

The recovery period following bunion surgery is as critical as any part of the operation, it is also the period where most patients feel somewhat isolated and not in control. It can be an unpredictable time as no two recoveries are the same, though advice will be given to you to try and ensure that there are as few surprises as possible. The recovery period is nevertheless the time when complications can develop.

Weight bearing

During the initial recovery period of the first two weeks after surgery, a surgical shoe will be fitted (Fig.4.1), which will accommodate the dressing but will also allow weight to be put on the foot, though usual advice will be to put weight on the heel and avoid too much weight being placed on the surgical site and ball of the foot.

Crutches & Rest

Crutches will also be provided to reduce the weight taken on the foot and give stability. In essence, the recovery period is when the patient needs to rest to allow the foot to heal with as little swelling as possible, but at the same time, it is important that mobilisation continues to reduce the risk of post-operative deep vein thrombosis. Most patients will be advised to sit with their foot elevated above the level of their hip but every 30 minutes' walk around the house. While sitting, it will also be helpful to pedal the foot up and down like you are on a bicycle. This activates the calf muscles to contract and squeeze the blood in the veins of the leg back towards the heart and lungs where it can be re-oxygenated and then once more returned to the circulation.

Failure to use the calf muscle pump can lead to failure of adequate blood flow, leading to the pooling of blood in the veins deep within the calf, which in turn will cause the blood to clot.

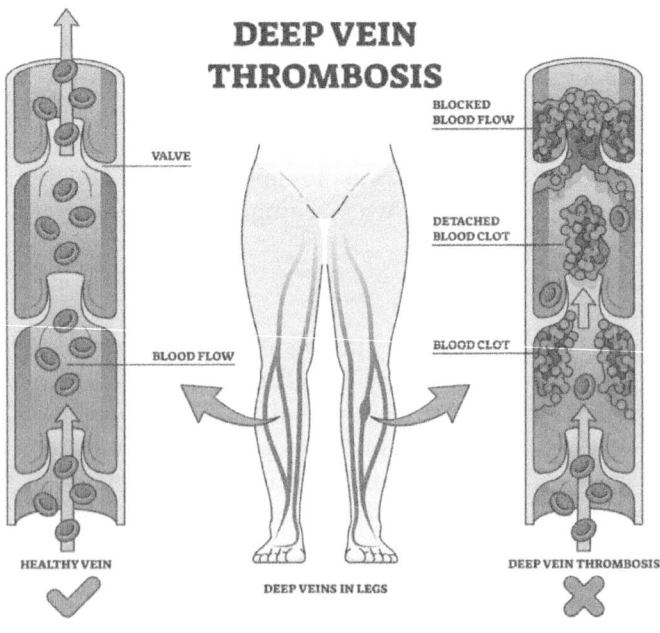

Fig.3.9. Showing valve backflow stagnation of red blood cells.

Blood Clot in the leg

The clot can block the vein Fig.3.9, and the normal passage of blood back to the heart, and then the leg will swell as the back pressure within the veins of the leg builds. Back pressure caused by the blockage will damage the valves within the veins of the legs, which can leave a lifetime problem of varicose veins. This is referred to as post-thrombotic syndrome, which has lifelong implications.

Early movement following the operation is an important way of reducing the risk of deep vein thrombosis, but the surgical team may also provide compression stockings and, in some cases, ask you to inject yourself with a blood thinner on the day of surgery and for several days or weeks after the surgery.

Pain control during the post-operative period will be planned by your surgical team. The critical period is the first three days and nights following surgery. Even though the foot may still be completely numb following the local anaesthetic nerve block, it is vital that the painkillers prescribed are taken at regular intervals. In this way the pain can be pre-empted and controlled much better as the analgesic levels within the patients system are usually sufficient to achieve this. Pain control can also be augmented by the use of ice. Ice will also help to reduce swelling, which is an important cause of pain. Excessive swelling can also lead to the opening of the wound. Figures 4.4 & 4.20 show alternative methods of cooling the foot after surgery.

Placing a bag of frozen peas or ice cubes on the front of the ankle, but not on the wound itself, for twenty minutes per hour every hour will also extend the effective analgesic effect—it is cheap and accessible.

Too much cooling, damage to the skin as in frost bit will delay wound healing and, as a consequence, increase the risk of wound infection.

Driving and Physical Activities

It may be possible to return to wearing trainers and some routine activities, including driving. Return to sport can, however, take between 8 and 12 weeks, but the patient is often the best judge as to when they should return to sport. If the foot is comfortable and swelling minimal there is no reason why sport should not be attempted. The best advice is to 'listen to what the foot is telling you.'

It is essential to bear in mind that everyone is different, and healing times vary. Optimum healing requires movement within reason. We have given a time frame of anything from 10 days to several weeks, but it is important to appreciate that deeper healing continues for months. Nerves and blood vessels repair slowly. Scar tissue fills in and then contracts, leading to reduced joint movement, and this is where physiotherapy is valuable—either using your own or attending a clinic. Bone takes longer to heal and consolidate. Swelling remains even months later, and this is not always abnormal, but patience is required.

Physiotherapy

Physiotherapy can help patients restore mobility, maintain functional joint movement, and diminish swelling. Sadly, little evidence exists for mandating physiotherapy, and not all orthopaedic or podiatric surgery departments offer this service. Consultants often play a lesser role following surgery but should be on hand to offer advice and support as needed.

Part III - Summary

The details of bunion surgery have been considered. While there are so many good reasons why someone undergoing bunion surgery should be aware of these issues, there is rarely sufficient time in a busy surgery department to discuss all these aspects of the operation and recovery. Even if time allowed, the volume of information would be overwhelming for most people.

No surgery is without risk; the best possible advice for someone contemplating surgery is that they should be aware of the risks and then balance those risks against the lifestyle limitations their bunion problem is causing them.

If the benefits of surgery outweigh the risks, then surgery has a lot to offer. Bunions are treatable, and the outcomes of surgery are on the whole excellent. There is really no justification in allowing the condition to reduce anyone's activity or lifestyle. Don't just take our word for this as clinicians and surgeons, read Part IV, where we allow patients to pick up the bunion story and share their surgical experiences. However, we warn you, not all stories have ended well.

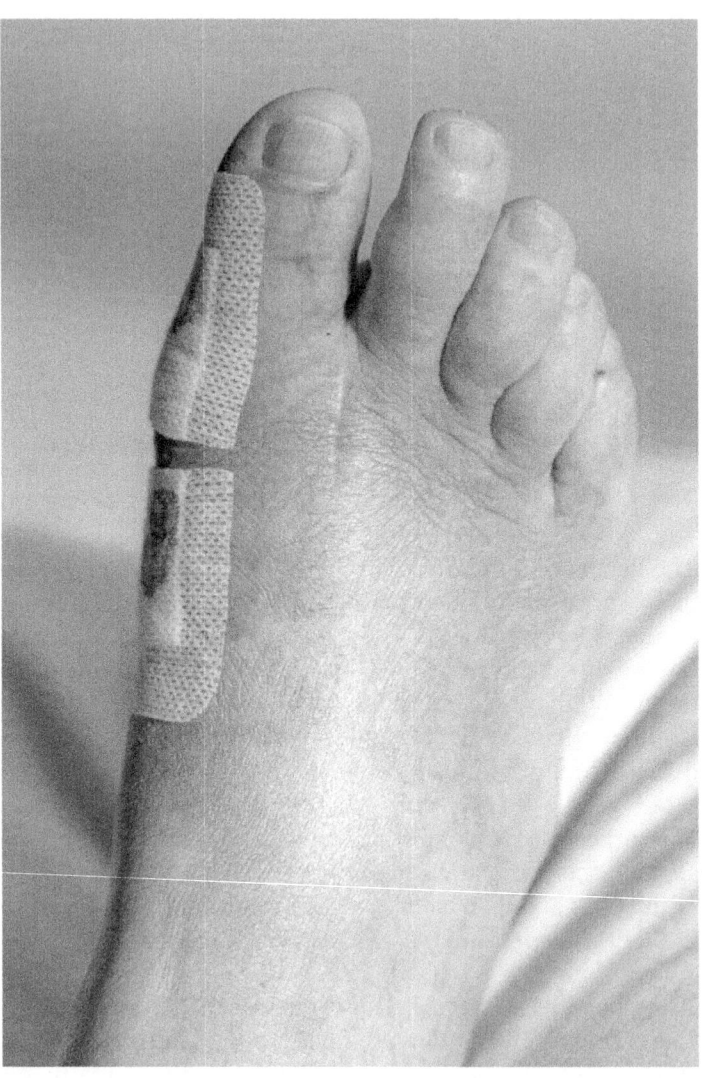

Fig. 3.10. Post operative dressings vary in size. The image shows a recent surgery with a scar just behind the interdigital cleft of the first and second toes. This informs us that this is most likely a revision surgery as the scar is mature. See Part IV for further post operative discussion

Part IV

No matter how well we counsel patients, our words can be misunderstood. As patients, our concentration wanes, and our ability to absorb complex information can degrade rapidly. Sometimes the information provided is overwhelming. Our hopes can encompass false expectations of a cure rather than an improvement.

Expectations are portrayed confidently, for the treating surgeon hardly wants to suggest *their* efforts will make you worse. During the period of the clinical consultation there will be a discussion covering the risks as well as the benefits of surgical treatment.

Relief from pain has always been our main objective and to create a return to full mobility. The narrative in these pages will open your eyes more than any consultation could hope. The index will be of value for specific topics, e.g. shower, pain, post-operative footwear, walker casts and driving.

Is there a best age for bunion surgery?

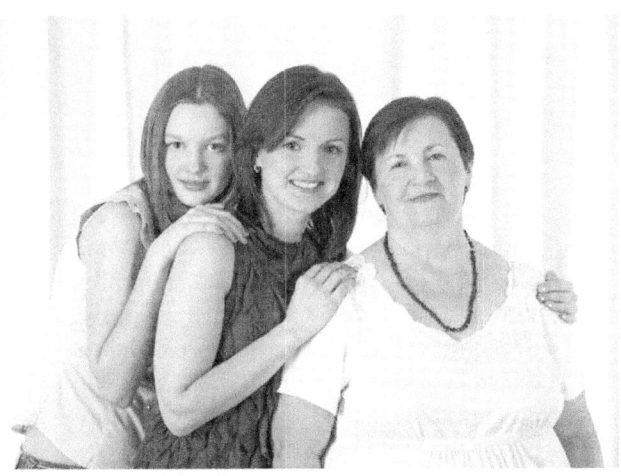

We might be obsessed with not having ugly feet like our grandparents or parents, but there is a right time and a wrong time to have surgery. While you can be operated on at any age, as a generalisation, 35-45 offers optimum results, lower risks, and greater optimism for success.

Bunion bump removal surgery (exostectomy) alone is never recommended in the presence of hallux valgus in younger, healthy, mobile, active patients. The short-term benefit and high recurrence from removing bumps make this undesirable.

Under Twenty

Babies can be born with a bunion, but this is rare and considered part of the pressure associated with the uterus; it is just as likely to have a club-shaped foot as a bunion.

The latter incidence is around 1 in 1000. The age of bone growth maturity is around 15-17 (girls) and 16-19 (boys). It is possible to have surgery and require a repeat not just once but twice. Our youngest patient was 14, but the most severe bunion was identified in a 9-year-old.

Children scar more readily than adults, which can add to concerns as scar lines thicken and are vivid and unsightly. Surgery at 14 may still lead to surgery at 20. The main justification for juvenile surgery (under 16) is for pain and recurrent damage to the skin with infection. Even surgery as an adult can see recurrence, albeit slower in progression. Revision surgery will be explored further in Part IV.

The Twenties

Recovery is excellent when young. Return to full function requires little rehabilitation, but skin scars may be unsightly. Recurrence of larger deformities arise, so long-term benefit into later life is not assured.

The Thirties

The deformity reoccurs slightly less after age 30-35 than in earlier years following surgery. Depending upon the source you read, there is a 7-15% reoccurrence risk. Bunion surgery is successful in 70-80% of cases, but about 20% of patients may not be as satisfied—

- Overcorrection (varus).
- Undercorrection – retained deformity.
- Increase in deformity.
- Pain problem.
- Prolonged footwear discomfort.
- Wound problems.

Starting a family after thirty+ is common today, especially

for those who have yet to settle down or have a significant career. Teachers have more challenges, especially if they have been pressured to return to school too early.

In another case, a 29 year old woman took three years for her joint to return to 60° of movement after surgery.

The Forties

Ages - 40-59 do well, although healing maybe slower. Pain control is effective if you follow all the ground rules. Of course, by now, the deformity might have increased, and those secondary features such as hammertoes, corns and a callus may have arisen. Combining surgery with other problems has to be considered, and recovery is extended than when younger. Bunion surgery is carried out more frequently between 40 and 65 than any other age. If your GP says your bunion is not ripe yet, *they* mean it is not severe enough for surgery. In the UK, this can often be a term to stop the NHS from overloading, where waiting lists are long.

Sixty Plus

Where sixty-year-olds remain active it is best to apply the same latitude to someone who wishes to remain active in good health. Our oldest patient was 94 and, while in good health, was troubled by damaged skin. Healing ability can drop, and the skin is more fragile, but post operative pain is better tolerated by many in this age group. Local anaesthetic is often more beneficial for the older patient, especially if their health is fragile. Simple surgery such as bump removal offers an advantage, restoring earlier mobility and independence. One of our concerns is ensuring patients have someone around to support their needs.

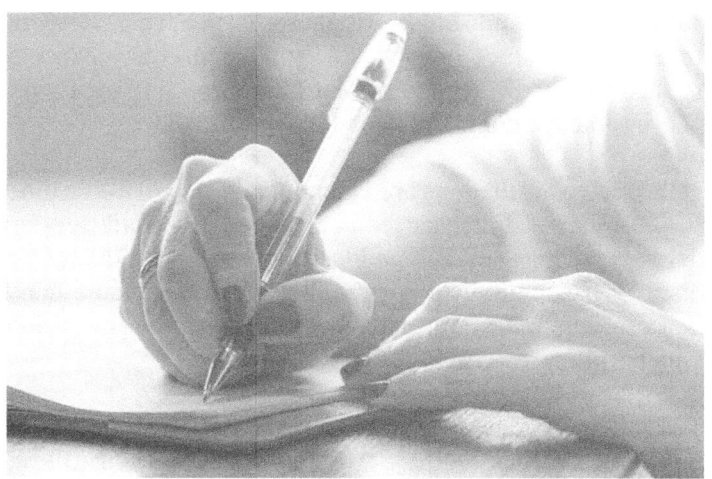

Biographical Stories after Surgery

These diaries offer rare insights into patient experiences after foot surgery. They are written mainly by patients who have undergone surgery. Both sides of the journey are shown to reveal the highs and lows. This makes each account unusual, as few books tell it as it is or was. Each story provides a slightly different perspective. Many stories demonstrate variations between patients despite similar procedures. Comments describe the hopes and disappointments within recovery. Dressing problems, managing at home, using creams on skin and the importance and effect of icing the foot throughout are covered.

Female patients reveal their need to undertake domestic chores rather than being able to rest—this often comes from lack of partner (usually male) support. A sense of boredom and a longing to return to normal are challenging for most patients. Not all journeys relate to those managed by the authors of this guide book. All photos used have been taken from licensed stock images and do not reflect any patients in this book. All pictures of feet have been provided with permission and complete knowledge of their use.

Unhurried consultations are essential and should allow time for questions. Clinicians focus on facts, time, safe service delivery, staying current, and learning new techniques. Our one big disappointment lies with the absence of more male diaries, although Tom relates his experience by interview, which sadly was largely negative.

The text has been edited for brevity while retaining critical milestones in each journey. After a brief entry from Alison, who informs us to pick the right time of year to have surgery, we continue with Jane, a podiatrist who has to come to terms with her experience on the other side of the clinical couch.

When to have Surgery?

Of all the testimonials received over the years, this one says much:

> Just wanted to say thanks for my new feet!! I'll look forward to showing them off in the summer. Thank you. Alison L (2007)

Winter offers a good opportunity because this leaves the summer to experience the benefit. However, not everyone believes this is the most convenient time. For example, shop owners find winter a busy time. It is worth reflecting when you might ideally prefer to have your surgery and plan that admission day with your foot surgeon. After all, optimal recovery may be dictated by the season. Of course, choice may be limited, but most surgeons try to accommodate as best they can.

Jane's Bunion Surgery[47] —clinician turned patient

Her own words

My bunion story starts nine years of age when my mother stopped me ballet dancing. I was just about to go 'en pointe', so I guess that would've made it even worse! Now, 50+ years later and as a *Silver Swan* (adult) ballet dancer, I now regret that I didn't pursue my dancing as a child, despite my mother's anxiety about my feet.

The Complaint

I have tolerated the 'bump' on the side of my foot for many years, and apart from early joint change pains, I can't say that it has troubled me greatly, apart from the obvious restriction of wearing certain shoes.

Having been a podiatrist for forty years, I have seen the consequences of my patients' bunions, some of whom have avoided surgical treatment and others who have had both

---

[47] Jane Clare was a practising podiatrist at the time of this publication. This story was written by Jane originally for the website ConsultingFootPain: Tales of Foot Surgery. (17 Sept 2021). This version has been edited for the book.

unsuccessful and successful procedures in the past. Over the last two years, I have noticed a deterioration of my foot condition with the progressively sideways displacement of my right big toe, causing the lesser toes to be pushed over into the sides of the footwear.

Seeking Help

Knowing the problems that can occur due to this pressure on the toes, I sought further advice from a foot and ankle specialist surgeon in 2020 for an initial consultation on the NHS. Initially, I would see him privately, but his secretary advised me that the X-ray/imaging fees would be quite costly.

As I had no pain/discomfort symptoms, a wait of a few months or more on the NHS would be acceptable. Of course, as my appointment was pre-Covid, I had yet to learn as to the extent of the waiting list looming. I had a follow-up appointment in September 2020 and was formally placed on the surgery waiting list and signed a consent form. I only had brief information given at this appointment and then assumed that I would have a long wait before seeing the surgeon again to discuss the procedure further. I had a phone call in March 2021 from the admissions at the County Hospital, offering me an earlier date for my surgery.

Work Considerations

Being a busy professional clinician with my patients booked weeks ahead, I had to decline the offer of imminent surgery and go 'back' on the waiting list as I couldn't organise everything quickly.

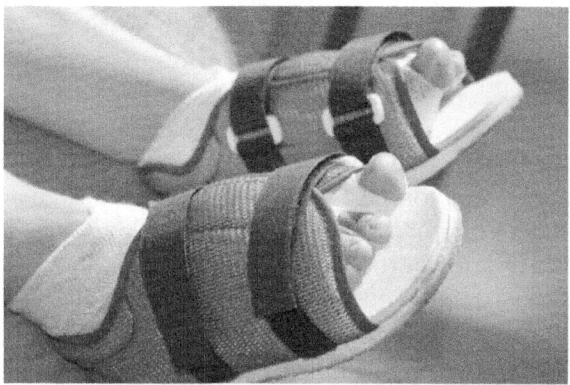

Fig.4.1 Post-operative shoes may not be glamorous but accommodate larger dressings comfortably.

The Day of Surgery

I was taken to the hospital at 7.30 in the morning of the operation, and following visits to my room by a multitude of staff for the next three hours, including the surgeon, I finally went into theatre at 10.40 am.

Everything went relatively smoothly, and I was surprised to awaken just after midday to find the operation was over and I saw a relatively straight alignment under the heavily bandaged elevated right foot. After a few hours in recovery, I was discharged home with a huge bag of painkillers and anticoagulant injections but no physiotherapy/Occupational therapy support. As I got dressed, I discovered a box with a shoe left on the shelf (Fig.4.1).

A nurse came to carry my bags and heel-walk me to my lift, waiting to take me home.

Left to my own devices

My experience overall was relatively good but I felt disinformed afterwards and wondered if this was due to the fact I was a podiatrist and that I should know it all. Over the next few days I gathered as much information as I could from books, podiatry friends and social media sites, and after a mass of conflicting opinions, came to the conclusion that I would just be sensible and use my common sense as to what worked for me and my foot. I was followed up at the hospital twice for re-dressing appointments and saw the surgeon briefly on both occasions. The elastic stocking[48] was advised for a further two weeks, but intolerance to discomfort, and as I had to take the anticoagulant injections for another four weeks, he gave in and said I could remove it.

My Experience

The whole 'bunion' corrective surgery was less complex than expected, relatively painless and much less burdensome. I would, therefore, recommend anyone contemplating surgery to go ahead as soon as possible. The younger and fitter you are, the quicker you are going to heal and re-mobilise. I was very fortunate that I knew the proficiency of my surgeon, I am relatively healthy and have fairly strong legs through walking a lot beforehand and my dancing of course.

---

[48] The elastic stocking was to reduce to risk of deep venous thrombosis.

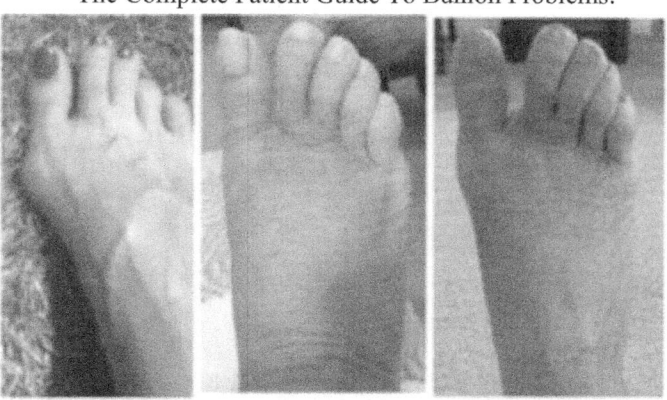

Fig. 4.2. Left to right: before, during recovery and after recovery
C/O Jane Clare

Pain Management

I probably have a stronger pain threshold than most, as I can honestly say my sleep, movement and activity have not been compromised too badly at all, but do not be deterred by horror stories of bunion operations. Medicine and surgery have moved on in leaps and bounds during the last ten years, and what was once a relatively complicated and disabling operation is now a straightforward, almost 'routine' procedure.

Three weeks after my operation, my foot appeared straighter, my wounds healed, and I even managed to take a short walk into the field outside our house today. I must add that I have been elevating my foot for most of the past eighteen days, and my numb posterior is a testament to that!

I hope everyone's experience and outcome are as satisfactory as mine. Remember that common sense must prevail, and if you're patient, good results will appear!

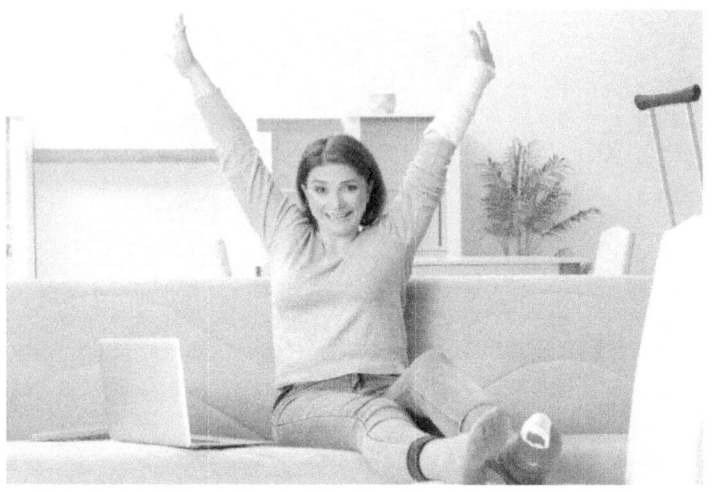

From the NHS to the independent (private) sector, with Jo.

Jo's Bunion Surgery – ex-nurse

Jo believed in the importance of good foot health and described her patient journey. These words are Jo's—

> I have suffered from a bunion for approximately 15 years. More recently, I have asked various medical people. Nothing constructive was offered so I limped on, walking on the outside of my affected leg and suffering pain in the knee on that side as well. As a walker who enjoys 1 to 2 hours of walking daily, I became worried about what I was going to do. In the past five years, I have had two hip replacements, and I want to preserve them for as long as possible. You suddenly realise how important your feet are! Then, a friend recommended a different surgeon.

The whole passage, from the initial assessment to surgery and the aftercare, was well organised. The consultations were unhurried and there was plenty of time to ask questions. There were comprehensive fact sheets about the available operations, with all the pros and cons.

All went smoothly on the day of surgery and exactly as explained on the fact sheet. I was taken aback that I needed a replacement joint, but the joint was worn out, so there was no option. I was most impressed with the physiotherapist I saw three times postoperatively before they discharged me. Eight weeks later, I had my first two-hour walk. My knee no longer hurt, and I tried to do what the physiotherapists taught me.

CLINICIAN COMMENT

The surgeon will constantly be confronted with the question of whether a joint can be preserved with an osteotomy or whether we need to fuse (arthrodesis) a big toe, use an interposition module such as a silastic spacer, or even resurface the joint. Most judgement is taken once the foot and joint can be visualised at surgery. Discussing the chances of changing procedures before the day of admission is useful.

Leah's Story[49] - Damaged first toe joint – hallux rigidus

Leah had not had surgery before. She kept a log from 2018, which she sent to ConsultingFootPain during the first seven months of her recovery. This was reviewed three years later. Leah was provided with information before undergoing an arthrodesis to her toe. She was diagnosed with a marked loss of joint space between the bone ends. The surrounding surface had spurs or projections (osteophytes). Hallux rigidus, as the name suggests, is a rigid first toe but may not always have a valgus-angle greater than the customary range of deformity +15°.

> My left bunion was noted three years ago by my Australian family. They were astonished that I had not had it removed. The bunion was unsightly and limited my choice of footwear. The first signs had been three years earlier as the feet had become more uncomfortable. They ached after walking even in sturdy walking boots. High heels used for dancing hurt.

Leah tried different shoes and then drifted toward felt pressure pads and silicone spacers between her second and first toe.

> I arranged to have the operation and was surprised how quickly the appointment came, which I had to delay because of holiday plans. At this time, my right foot was becoming very painful over the big toe with arthritis.

---

[49] Leah's story (not her real name) was first published by ConsultingFootPain July 2021 and written by her with comments from the author DRT.

Due to a cancellation, I was able to have both feet done at the same time. I would highly recommend having both feet done together.

CLINICIAN COMMENT - Arthrodesis

While bunion surgery does not require fusion to make it stiff, if the joint is damaged, the surgeon is faced with trying to stop movement surgically, where conservative treatment fails. The use of night splints and stiff-soled shoes can help. A female patient passionate about shoes with heels must be aware that once a joint is fixed, the height of a shoe is determined by the position of the toe afterwards. This position is usually elevated by 5-10°, so the toe is deliberately placed slightly off the ground.

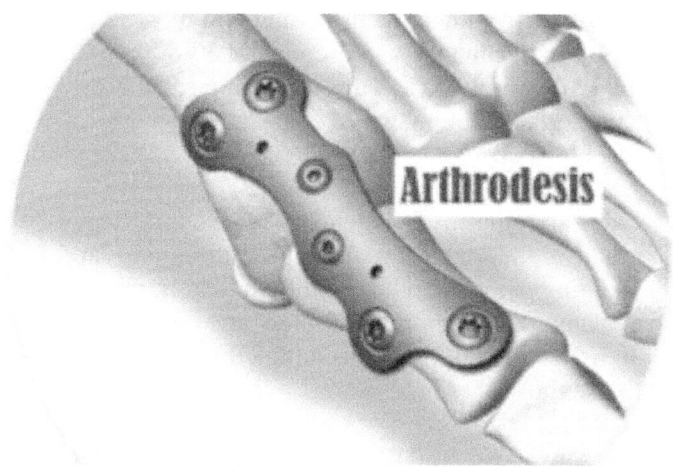

Fig.4.3. Arthrodesis—a plate ensures the joint no longer moves and bonds at the point of the former joint. Pins and screws may still be used.

Leah's surgery was performed under local anaesthetic. Leah continues describing being in theatre:—

In theatre a screen was placed in front of me - a calm atmosphere was helped with soothing music and constant reassurance from the staff. I managed to read two chapters of my book. There was no feeling in my feet during the operation, just the sound of the saw and drill. It was all over in less than an hour. I felt calm knowing what to expect and told the anaesthetic could last up to 10 hours.

Around 6.45 pm I started to feel the anaesthetic wearing off with some throbbing and by 7.30 pm I took two pain tablets (co-codamol 30-500mg) as the pain was intense. I tried watching the World Cup for distraction whilst lying in bed with my feet elevated.

I kept moving my legs which seemed very heavy to ease the pain. I experienced throbbing and shooting pains in both feet so tried to keep my feet elevated. I took more painkillers at 11.30 pm and an hour later felt nauseous with a dread of having to use the bathroom.

I was awake at 5.30 the next morning and my feet were not throbbing so much but still painful. I had a bedside wash and cuppa tea then took 1 tablet at 7.30 am. Again I felt a little nausea but the pain was controlled. I noticed a tiny area of blood on my big toe. A bit of elevation helped using two pillows.

Day one - Leah slept during the morning of her first day after surgery and developed shooting pains on top of her right foot in the afternoon. A single painkiller worked. Nearly six hours later, the throbbing started again, so she found that taking the pain medication worked up to its maximum (six-hour) benefit. She could wiggle her toes and had a shower with plastic bags. As this was June, she spent an hour in the sun. She was even walking without crutches using casts.

One week+ Leah required no additional pain control and felt she could stand on her feet without wincing. Sleep had improved, and she used pain medication sparingly when the feet throbbed, usually in the evening. Her legs were often recorded as feeling tired and heavy. By twelve days, she was managing a shower and washing her hair while sitting on a stool again with plastic bags as her feet still had dressings. Her feet tended to throb at bedtime, but she did not need pain medication. The next day, she found the hot weather caused her restlessness, and she had to be careful not to walk too much. Her check-up was at the two-week mark.

Two weeks -The casts used on her feet were removed using a cast cutter. These caused a little anxiety, but the noise was scarier than the actual cutter, which only vibrates and is safe from cutting the skin.

> Everyone was pleased with the healing process. I was then able to wear trainers and told to walk 'flatfooted' with most of the pressure on the heels. The next appointment was in five weeks.

Her feet felt a lot cooler without the casts, which allowed her to start massaging the scar and bathe the foot. She was able to moisturise the foot, which helped remove some of the dead skin that makes the enclosed foot flaky.
The foot had ankle swelling and was bruised on the balls of her foot and one of her toes. The trainers had to be used

without laces; otherwise, it would have been tender over the scars where the incision had been made. By two weeks, Leah was more comfortable. She was showering and finding massaging around the scars manageable and using Bio-oil. The skin tapes (steristrips) were no longer required, any swelling in her left foot had diminished, and the bruising had faded. The swelling persisted around the scar area. Walking was still limited around the house for short periods. Swelling increased when overused. At night, there was occasional stabbing pain over the left bunion. She noted that she missed walks and dancing, and keep-fit classes.

Three—four weeks - Leah could walk to the end of her street, which was about 100 yards, 'quite easily'. Her left big toe ached in the evening. Now that her operation was nearly four weeks old, she started to walk *comfortably around town using sandals mostly.*' She was driven to the shops.

The swelling was still present, and the scar was faintly pink, which she maintained with Bio-oil daily. Her walking was slower than normal.

Five—six weeks - Her legs and feet were tired after a walk around the shops. She pointed out that her feet swelled up in the wrong shoes. Tenderness over the scar area was helped by purchasing some wider shoes. She noted that her big toes tended to bend slightly toward the next toe, and swelling persisted around the scar area. Massage was to be maintained. Leah was fortunate, as she had retired and was able to swim, cycle, and do a little line dancing.

I love walking but find my feet ache so the distance is limited. Trainers and Velcro fastening sandals though my Havana's flip flops are comfortable around the house, they also help to keep a space between the big toes.

Past the 2-month mark - Today, her problem centred around her big toes rubbing. She had a painful ball of her right foot under her big toe due to wearing the wrong shoes. She felt she needed a lot of cushioning under the sole, so she went back to her trainers. This did not put her off, and she embarked on travelling around the coast.

Some aching side of the balls of my feet and under my big toes. Enjoyed some walking and line dancing. Scars are so faint, very pleased with the whole operation.

Her next entry showed that her feet and accustomed changes altered frequently.

Feet are comfortable but the first toes are raised around their joints causing some friction in some shoes. My flip flops are the most comfortable around the house. This week I wore kitten heels comfortably. My friend has decided to have her bunion done she is so impressed with my surgery.

Three months - 'Nearly invisible scars,' were noted. The only problem was her left big toe rubbing the toe next to it. She used an inexpensive silicone toe cap that was comfortable when wearing closed shoes and was back to Line Dancing. Raising her spirits she booked a break in Spain.

Lots of walking just about forgot I had the bunions done wore sandals flip flops high heels dancing, No problems, Pretty Feet!! Continue to massage and moisturise very night. Back home now and in regular footwear - some big toe discomfort in certain shoes and boots better in my widest sizes. I find my toes don't like the fit of opaque tights. The big toes tend to rub the second toes. I think my feet prefer sandals.

Then she developed chilblains (November)! Of course, it is easy to create this if sandals are used in cold weather. She recorded 'itchy painful thin skin over the big toes...' The chilblains lasted one week, and she thought this was caused by the hot water bottle and walking around London shopping.

A recurrent problem associated with big toes pushing against the second toe kept being recorded, as well as 'finding my toes ache unless I wear cushion or memory soles.' Leah was followed up in mid-December and had another X-ray and readying herself to go abroad in 2019 on a long-haul flight. She flew out in the new year, and in February 2019, seven months after surgery, she records in her 'bunion diary'.

Hi, I'm just back from Australia. My feet are okay for cycling, hiking, and swimming. I had my assessment in December with photos. The only problem is that both big toes lean and rub the second toe, making the skin break (not good as I have diabetes type 2). I use gel toe protectors to stop the rubbing.

By 2020, the UK was hit with the pandemic, and so we followed up with Leah in April 2021, just under three years after her original surgery in 2018. Her response by e-mail was encouraging. We asked whether she had any setbacks since surgery.

> I need to use silicone toe spacers between the big toes and both feet. Otherwise, the big toe rubs the next toe until it is very sore. The first toes both have some arthritis no pain. The procedure was successful. The only problem re diabetes is cold feet in bed. I can wear any shoe, Yes I would have the procedure again both feet at the same time. I can pursue my usual activities; line dancing, keeps fit, class, cycling, rambling, club gardening. I have beautiful feet now.

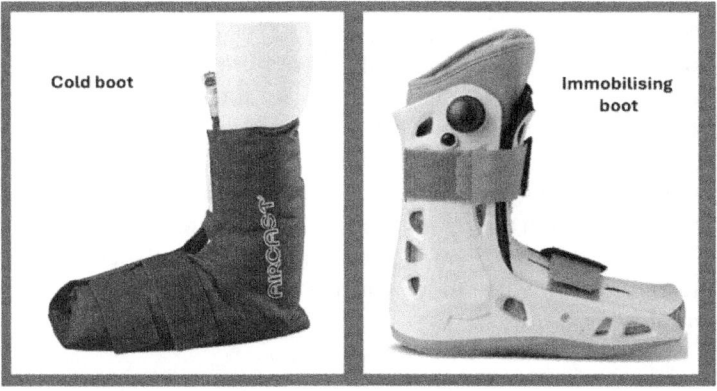

Fig.4.4 Cold Cryotherapy boots and Aircast™ immobilising boots allow controlled walking, safety from protection, and the ability to return to many activities sooner.

Scar Management

As clinicians, we learn as much from patients as we do from working within multidisciplinary teams. Impressed with one physiotherapist's approach to scars, a new philosophy was implemented.

> Good scar management can enhance healing and speed recovery.

Creams can make a difference when applied. The video[50], produced by a BMI hospital and tissue nurse, offers additional information. Although it does not show feet, the principles remain the same. The video, on YouTube is called Scar Management Guide (5.54m) 2013.

Scars can take several years to reduce. The purpose of reducing the bulk of scar tissue made of excess fibrous tissue is to break this down as quickly as possible. Too much scar around the first mtpj reduces toe movement. Excessive scarring can tether nerves, causing pins and needles, shooting pain, and tenderness. Massage reduces this risk. Keloid is as likely in white, pale skin as it is in black, coloured skin, despite general literature suggesting an increase in black skin. Patients under twenty can produce more scar tissue as repair is often faster after injury.

---

[50] https://video.search.yahoo.com/search/video?fr=aaplw&ei=utf-8&p=scar+management+after+surgery#id=1&vid=8cab4262114ba635b4f6948dffb3defe&action=click. Accessed September 2024.

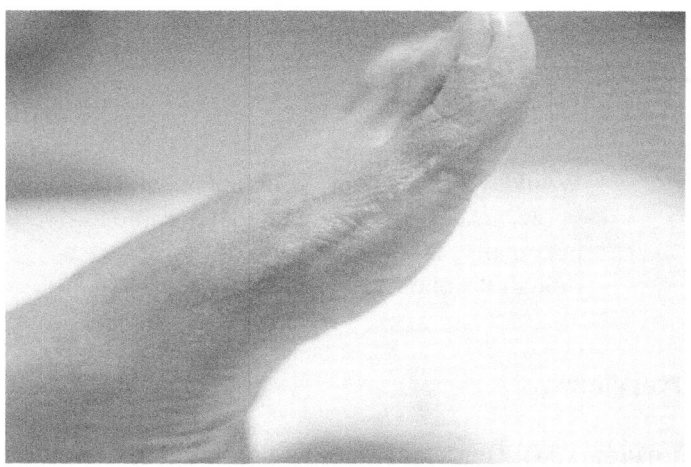

Fig. 4.5. A typical scar following surgery with mild thickening and around three months following surgery. Source: Shutterstock. Asian girl.

When To Massage?

The wound should not be open, nor should the skin be infected. Start gently pressing down when using circular motions. Build the pressure and repeat it several times daily.

Initially, there is a reluctance to put pressure on a tender area of the foot. Push the tissue back as well to reduce congestion and local swelling. This will bring new blood, oxygen, and nutrients to the site while helping drain back through the lymphatic channels.

How Long To Massage?

Massage until the wound is flat, no longer tender, and has no tingling sensations. This may be six weeks and, in some cases, longer. A deeper scar should continue to be massaged until the joint is more flexible.

Florinda, Jackie And Rose – Hallux Valgus deformity correction

> Would I do it again, knowing what I know now? Yes, I would, but for me personally, it's been a difficult journey, though it's one worth taking. *Jackie*

Overview

Florinda (34) Her chief complaint during the surgical period included resistance to her pain medication, constipation and piles. Florinda was an active woman and had a husband to support her surgery, but nevertheless, the thought of surgery was daunting, and the idea of being laid off her feet filled her with some dread. She explains the emotional side of surgery and the effects of constipation leading to the less glamorous complication of piles. She tells us that:

I have had a bunion deformity on my left foot since my adolescence, a hereditary deformity over time that became unbearably painful. The last two years I have been in agonising pain with normal activities such as walking and fitness classes and kneeling down becoming more difficult. The decision to have surgery was taken early in 2017 and involved an osteotomy to sort out the joint on my left foot bunion.

Jackie (46) had surgery previously on her other foot eight months before and had done well. She tried conservative steroid injections three times before electing for more surgery. Jackie's diary covers the six months following surgery and describes her second journey. She explains her thoughts, concerns, fears and attitude to conservative management. Her decision was far from cosmetic, and her story emphasises that recovery is not always straightforward.

Her account covers a wound complication, wrestling with pain medication that did not suit her. The curious part of her story relates to pain at the site of her original surgery affecting the opposite foot. This allows us to consider the effect of surgery on both feet.

One Foot Or Two Feet?

One unanswered question is whether we should have both feet operated on at the same time or tackle each foot separately. There is no hard and fast rule for this, and it must be for the consultant and patient to consider each aspect. Mobility, pain, length of surgical recovery and type of anaesthetic are some considerations that might be debated.

Rose (69) also had surgery before and came back to have her other foot managed. Her family had grown up, and there are many lovely relationship comments. She covers issues such as how to fit parties in, especially at Christmas, cook, go to the hairdressers and walk dogs—no surprises who had problems afterwards. Rose continued up to the fifth week after surgery and married her partner in the summer of 2018 without any undue consequences from her foot.

Rationale for Surgery

Jackie: After putting off bunion surgery for over a decade, steroid injections gave her some quality of life, but the relief was short-lived and lasted just a few months. She had a good support network around her, which would make the operation more manageable. With four children and two dogs, life was hectic. She aimed to be pain-free.

Experience From Previous Surgery

Jackie: My right foot had always given me the most pain, so I decided to do that first. My surgery went well, and I had one screw fitted. My wound healed quickly. I had several 'physio' sessions, which helped. Driving was the only thing I was anxious about, and I think this was more psychological than anything else. I eventually drove after eight weeks. Things were going very well, but three months in, I became complacent and jet-washed the patio, resulting in the jet-wash machine falling onto my operated toe. This set me back, but fortunately, everything was fine, and I just had bruising. Following my first operation, I decided to wait another five months before I had the other foot done. I wanted to enjoy the school summer holidays, get our youngest started at high school, and settle two of our teenagers at university. To enable me to do this, I opted to have a third steroid injection into my left foot so that I could be pain-free while waiting. This worked well for a few weeks, but the pain did return, reaffirming that I was doing the right thing in having the second surgery.

Day of surgery (Day Zero)

Florinda: I came round from the (general) anaesthetic and was starving. I knew the trick to make sure I didn't suffer from complications such as constipation, which relied upon a good diet and plenty of fluids. Unfortunately, this still wasn't going to be the case. The morphine[51] and co-dydramol I was given caused havoc with my stomach, causing me to spend the night after surgery [in hospital] awake with stomach cramps. By 6.30 the next morning, I was washed, dressed and packed, ready to go home.

Jackie: While I waited to be sent for, I took the opportunity to do my online grocery shop, as this had proved invaluable the first time around. By mid-morning, I was taken to the theatre, where everyone made me feel relaxed and at ease.

Back from theatre: The recovery staff were very friendly; all had gone well, and I'd got two screws in my toe. A cryotherapy cuff (Fig. 4.4) covered my foot, and I could feel no pain – due to an ankle block. I was taken back to the ward. A nurse helped, with the aid of crutches, to go to the 'loo'—*bathroom*. When I had the first operation, I found this aspect particularly challenging as my coordination wasn't great – but with practice, this became easier.

Jackie was discharged late afternoon as a day surgery patient and used a wheel chair to the car. Armed with a special shoe until my Aircast™ boot (Fig.4.4) was fitted at the first dressing change appointment. I took away a cryotherapy cuff, a pair of crutches and a Limbo cover (Fig.4.5), together with those all-important pain medications. Jackie's parents supported her during the daytime.

---

[51] Morphine is an opioid pain killer and accounts for many post-surgical problems. The need for morphine is lessened by using a good anaesthetic block.

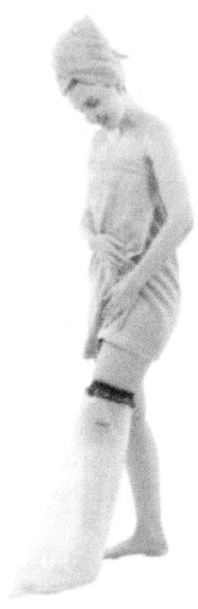

Fig.4.6. Limbo Cover for the leg and foot, invaluable for safe showering while retaining the dressing.

Mobility After Surgery

At home I elevated my feet and took my first dose of pain relief medication, although I was in absolutely no pain at this point. The pharmacist had stressed how important it was to stay on top of the pain control. This certainly worked first time around, so I was happy to do it again. The evening was spent on the sofa, and I was able to get to the downstairs toilet wearing the provided shoe, my trainer on the good foot and using the crutches. After my first operation, getting up the stairs for the first time was a huge issue, but this time, I managed to get up quite easily by shuffling up on my bottom without putting any weight on my left foot.

Rose: Having had the same procedure before, I was at least aware of what to expect. It was only necessary to remove the gel nail varnish from my left index finger; for ladies, this is useful information. The physiotherapist went over my exercises, the anaesthetist explained what she would be doing and the surgeon marked my foot with a large arrow. I was able to heel walk, with the aid of a crutch, to the bathroom.

The surgeon popped by to chat and show me a photo he had taken of my damaged cartilage – very graphic. The surgeon told me earlier to ice around the hindfoot rather than directly on the wounded area.

After a five-minute drive home, I settled down with my foot up and an Aircast ice boot on. The dressing boot was rather large as my foot is small, and my foot was not in contact with the boot, so I put a bag of frozen peas under my heel inside the boot, which made it more comfortable and gave an ice boost. I enjoyed a tasty meal cooked by my partner under instructions from my chair. He was being quite amiable – I didn't know how long it would last as he was not a tolerant soul at the best of times, although his mood would vary. As my foot was still numb, I was feeling no pain, so painkillers were not needed; I did, however, take one ibuprofen (for the anti-inflammatory benefit) before going to bed at 10 pm, with a couple of shoe boxes to raise the duvet and keep the weight off my foot. Apart from a couple of visits to the bathroom, I had a good night's sleep. I tackled the stairs on my bottom, which I found safest.

DAY 1

Florinda: The lack of sleep (*Florrie remained in the hospital overnight*) and being away from my five-year-old was very emotional. So when the surgeon phoned to check on me I had a meltdown with lots of tears.

Emotion—I cried with exhaustion. Still it took my mind off the foot, which was still quite numb but with a dull throb. The morphine and co-dydramol were exchanged for paracetamol and ibuprofen. After discharge home mid-morning I settled myself onto the sofa with the cryotherapy boot attached and plenty of ice. Unfortunately, I found this rather cumbersome and found using normal ice packs much more comfortable. Lack of sleep from the previous night meant that I napped the afternoon away. My main stance was maintaining a routine to keep my sanity.

Jackie: Oh, dear, I had no sleep whatsoever, which is very unusual for me. I was not in any pain though; I just couldn't switch off. At 11.30 am I noticed a pins and needles sensation in my foot so the ankle block must be wearing off. I started to use the cryotherapy [ice] cuff (Fig.4.4) during the evening. The moderate but bearable pain soon subsided with more pain control.

Rose: I woke at around 8 am feeling refreshed. My foot felt warmer than when I went to bed, so I guessed the local anaesthetic had worn off as I had a slight tingling on the top of the foot. I took two 500mg paracetamol with breakfast. I sat in the bath dangling my leg over the edge. Another hour later, while returning from my bathroom, I noticed that blood was seeping through the bandage underneath my big toe, and the top of my foot was sore and tingling. I sat for the next four hours with my foot raised above hip level. Thankfully, the bleeding stopped, and the pain lessened. Another dose of paracetamol and one 400mg ibuprofen at lunch while I remained sitting with my foot raised. Late afternoon I tackled the stairs on my bottom, which I found safest and easiest as our stairs are curved. The pain was greater than mild, but not severe. At dinner I took more 500mg paracetamol and ibuprofen and retired at 10 pm feeling rather groggy and miserable. The local anaesthetic had certainly worn off.

CLINICIAN COMMENT - sleep

Day surgery offers the advantage of sleeping in your own bed. Hospitals, even with private rooms, are not entirely comfortable because of disturbance and regular monitoring by nursing staff. Most bunion surgery can be performed in daycare, but discharge to responsible home care is essential.

DAYS 2–4

Florinda: The first night passed uneventfully – I slept well with no problems. I had only throbbing pain, which was managed with naproxen, previously prescribed, and an alternative to paracetamol. Getting up and down the stairs took more effort as the safest option was to go up and down on my bottom, much to the amusement of my five-year-old. Showering meant climbing into the bath and sitting down to shower with my operated side resting on the bath. After experiencing this for the first time, I would certainly have more empathy for my patients, who are usually advised to keep their dressings on and dry. I was given a Limbo cover (Fig.4.6) to use in the shower. However, I was able to safely sit in the bath and shower so had no use for it.

Jackie: After a wonderful night's sleep I woke up in quite strong pain and again this eased once the painkillers kicked in. I elevated [my leg] and intermittently iced with the cryo cuff for most of the day, so the pain was kept well under control. Day 3 had probably been the worst for pain but by Day 4, I slept well again and managed to spread out the time between doses of painkillers.

I wanted to take a shower but felt very dizzy, probably as a result of the drugs I was using. Washing at the basin was exhausting.

Rose: Feeling a bit brighter – not using the toilet during the night helped. The throbbing and tingling sensation had eased a little, and I felt comfortable. I took paracetamol with breakfast, then hobbled to the bathroom to wash, but not to take a bath again. I have managed to negotiate walking with one crutch, and a hop allowed me to keep my injured foot off the ground entirely. I decided to wait a few more days before attempting to heel walk again as I didn't want a recurrence of a bleed. Spent all morning watching TV and doing crosswords. At 1.30 pm finding the pain moderate so took another paracetamol.

Pain eased by late afternoon, and it was good to sit at the dining table for a change, as opposed to using a tray on my lap, then back to an easy chair with my foot elevated and iced with frozen peas. That evening I started to feel uncomfortable, tired and fidgety, probably a result of sitting all day with no exercise, so I made my way to bed early. It is far easier going down on one's bottom than going up – it puts a lot of strain on arms, but on the positive side, it's good exercise for the pectoral muscles. I found it easier than negotiating curved stairs with a crutch.

Day 3 - I used one paracetamol as a precaution, as the pain was mild to moderate. On Day 4, the dressing was changed.

Feeling Faint At Redressing

I asked to lie flat on the couch as previously, when the first dressing came off, I felt a little faint – fear of not knowing what to expect – so I was taking no chances this time as I knew what I would see. However, the dressing came off without a hitch, although some dried blood made it stick to the wound, but it caused no pain on removal.

The nurse pointed out two large blood blisters on the top of my foot under the Steristrips, so she left them uncovered. There had been quite a lot of soreness and discomfort in this area so I guess these were the culprits. It would be interesting to see if they disappeared when the dressing was changed again. Once the wound was cleaned, it looked much neater than the right foot, which had been operated on eleven months before.

DAYS 5–12

Florinda: Day 5 with the nurse for my dressing change. I was frightened. Thankfully, everything was OK, and I was able to look at my foot and check for myself. The dressing was changed, and I was allowed an Aircast boot (Fig.4.4) and one crutch. This allowed me to put my foot to the ground; a joyous moment so that I literally skipped and hobble-skipped out of clinic. With my Aircast I felt I had more freedom to get out and about. With the festive period [Christmas] in full swing I had invitations from friends to take me out for coffee to get me out of the house.

The next few days passed with me walking and doing tasks around the house with my Aircast boot on. I would feel the effect if I had been on the foot for an hour and experienced a heavy sensation that appeared very swollen. This was my cue to stop doing whatever I was doing and rest and elevate it. The pain was negligible by this point without the need for pain relief on a regular basis, and then only paracetamol or ibuprofen as required, i.e. when I had overdone things. I ventured out, which helped with my mental well-being, and my Aircast caused great interest.

Jackie: My first dressings were changed at Day 5 – the grand reveal. Unfortunately, I was feeling sick and dizzy, so the nurse and house doctor (Resident Medical Officer) checked my observations because of the dizziness, but they were all fine.

I do not tolerate certain pain tablets very well, so I had a feeling it might be them. I was pleased with how the wound looked and there was absolutely no pain when having the bandages removed. The Aircast boot allowed me to get around the house a little, but I noticed some blood seeping through the dressing. I managed without pain control until night-time.

Day 8 - I was pain-free, and the vertigo feeling seemed to have abated. I felt confident enough to shower with the Limbo cover on. Putting the Limbo on was not easy, and I had to have help, but once on, I could take a quick shower and my leg and foot remained completely dry. I felt wiped out after the shower but much better for it. A day later I was quite fed up, low and emotional, but my spirits were lifted as my son arrived home from university for a couple of days.

Jackie had had her other foot operated on five months previously, and now this started to ache. She put this down to having to take the burden of greater weight. Problems appeared at nine days following surgery.

Wound Problems & Delayed Healing

I awoke in pain, reluctant to take tablets, as I felt so much better without them, and I was concerned, having seen a darkened blood stain on the dressing, which wasn't due to be changed at the hospital for another seven days. The pain increased as the day progressed, and I was worried that there was an infection.

I managed to get an appointment with a nurse at my local GP surgery, thinking that it was best to get it checked as it was a Friday, and I didn't want it to worsen over the weekend.

Now a stone heavier than when I had the first surgery, I walked to the nurse's department on crutches and noticed the extra effort. I wasn't overweight when I had the first surgery but I did make a conscious effort to lose a few pounds prior to it. The wound was still bleeding and the bruising had started to come out but there appeared to be no infection so she redressed it and made an appointment for me to have it dressed again two days later. I was happy to get home and elevate my foot and reluctantly took my pain medication as advised, but even then the pain didn't fully disappear. At least I was able to get a good night's sleep.

Day 12 - another GP appointment and dressing change. When the nurse removed the dressing I was quite shocked as the wound was completely wet, the flesh had gone a dreadful colour and was oozing with blood, and there were also several blisters. Fortunately, it wasn't infected (my worst fear) and the nurse thought that the last type of dressing had caused the area to sweat. I'd also been wearing some very warm thick fluffy socks and I wonder if this had contributed. The nurse cleaned the wound, applied some Inadine [iodine] gauze and redressed the foot with a breathable dressing as applied originally by the hospital. I didn't feel like going straight home, so my friend drove us to a local supermarket for a coffee. I sat with my leg elevated the whole time.

Normally I could sit and chat with my friend for hours but today I was exhausted and in pain so we went home after 30 minutes. I got home, took some painkillers and spent the rest of the day resting on the sofa as it would be silly to make it worse and take me longer to recover in the long run if I pushed myself too much now.

Rose: (*Her first week*) I have mastered the art of getting in and out of the bath keeping my left leg clear of the water – being nimble and agile had its advantages. No pain on waking, but after bathing and dressing and manoeuvring downstairs, I felt uncomfortable. I felt better with my foot elevated and a pack of frozen peas under the heel/arch of my foot. No need for any medication today but shooting pain from my toes and across the top of my foot lasted a few minutes and was quite painful, which made me 'ouch' out loud.

My partner dropped me off at the door to my hairdressers, which was literally five minutes' drive away. I heel-walked with a post-op shoe and crutches about two metres to the salon's door, which wasn't a problem, and it was nice to be pampered. Every day now, I feel a little more human. There was no pain, so there were no tablets, but after having left off the medication for three days, my bowels returned to normal and I felt more comfortable.

I had got used to the 'usual' shooting pains today and a slight throbbing on the underside of the big toe that came and went. It's exactly a week since my operation, and it seems to have been a long week, but I do feel that I am now well on the road to recovery. Overall, my foot didn't feel as swollen as the previous foot did at this stage, so I was optimistic that it wouldn't take as long to return to normal. My other foot took 9–10 months to return to normal completely.

Heartburn played up, so I took some medication and sat up in bed to wait for it to ease. Overall I was better on waking and the shooting pains I had experienced were less frequent. The foot didn't look swollen, as much as I could tell through the bandages, but it felt as though the strips holding the wound together were tight. I thought maybe it was time for the bandages and strips to come off and let some air get to the wound. I decided to ring the outpatients department and see what they suggested.

I sat with my leg elevated and applied ice to try and relieve the pressure. I found it frustrating not being able to do anything, but it would be worth it at the end of the day. I continued to sit with foot elevated and iced and only used my heel when I walked to the toilet, consequently my right hip seemed aggravated due to extra strain being put on it. I carried out my exercises diligently but the cycling exercise made the muscles in my groin ache. I felt I was trying my best to be the 'perfect patient'. The sore, pulling, pressure sensation from yesterday had eased but my appointment couldn't come quick enough to have the dressings removed and a lighter dressing applied (See Fig.3.10).

Day 12 - The pulling/pressure sensations had dwindled, but when I climbed into bed last night, the sharp shooting pains returned with a vengeance and lasted for a good 15 minutes. After this, I had a good night's sleep. One more day to go until the bandages come off. Occasional stinging in the wound area with shooting pains from the big toe but on a scale of 1–10, maximum discomfort would rate at 3. My partner is getting short-tempered now, having to cook, clean and do the laundry – his level of attentiveness has rapidly diminished, so I need to get mobile soon!

DAYS 13–30

Florinda: I was advised the sticky tapes called Steristrips could come off in the next few days whilst in the shower. The surgery site had scabbed over nicely. There was still some swelling but nothing severe, and by this point, I was taking no pain relief but still using the Aircast boot and one crutch to walk with. There was a small opening which was still weeping, so I dressed it with sterile gauze and this soon dried up after a couple of days.

I had a lot of peeling dry skin on the operated foot as I was still keeping the foot out of the bath and only washed it once. I had completed the rest of my shower so that nothing was contaminating the wound site. I developed piles from lack of activity and the co-dydramol.[52] After a fretful few days thinking that I had bowel cancer my GP put my mind at rest. I decided I needed to be more active to improve my condition and to stop me feeling depressed, but experienced no foot pain after exercising and have had no pain since day 19. Some days the foot was more purple and swollen but improved with rest. There is no pain, even with a few minor mishaps such as a clumsy five-year-old stepping on my operated foot.

The first physiotherapy session, at four weeks, went well with advice covering re-introduction of 'normal' footwear gradually and commencing weight bearing on the operated foot. I elected to use trainers to accommodate the swelling. My operated foot was massaged and manipulated, which felt amazing as it was the first time that I felt normal sensation return to my foot. Strangely I had been too scared to touch my foot myself. Weight-bearing was attempted today (Day 29) when getting out of bed without crutches or my Aircast so I walked unaided for the first time. It felt strange and my walking pattern had naturally altered. Most importantly there was no pain. The surgery site continued to heal well with the established scab starting to lift away. I have limited feeling around the incision site; however, when it is touched, which I try to avoid, there is a strange sensation of pins and needles.

Jackie: (*Her delayed healing*) I started to worry as I could see the wound had seeped through the dressing again at Day 13. I generally didn't feel at all well and the pain seemed to build progressively as the day went on. My husband took me to our local (NHS) hospital in the evening for them to take a look.

---

[52] Codydramol contains codeine and is renowned to cause constipation.

When the nurse removed the dressing it looked so much better than yesterday but was still quite wet in one area where one of the blisters had burst. The nurse redressed the wound and said that it would be okay to leave for two days now, coinciding with my two-week checkup at my original hospital. I managed without painkillers during the day but took some at night. My wound had leaked through the dressing but just in the area where the blister had burst.

At my next appointment I was pleased as I thought I was getting back on track, although the blister still oozed a little. The wound was redressed, and another check booked in four days. The blister felt very sore due to the Aircast boot rubbing the area, so I rested the foot as much as possible to promote healing.

Day 16/17 - I needed pain relief at after waking in terrible pain at 3 am and then returned to a very sound sleep. I don't remember needing pain relief for this long first time around, but my wound healed much more quickly. However, by Day 18, I felt refreshed, able to cook a full English breakfast for the family and did a few light chores. I knew my limitations though; my foot felt incredibly heavy and tingly, and the wound area would become sore. Trying to take it easy we went to my in-laws for our evening meal and rested my foot for the whole time we were there. Today was definitely my best day so far. A small weeping area had leaked through by the time we got home. But, I could shower now without the Limbo – I was overjoyed. Turned a corner and managed the night without pain relief.

Day 21 - my foot had improved, and the nurse was happy for me to leave the dressing off but to cover with a gel bunion guard. I had a pain-free night.

Day 23 - it was great to be doing something different and after a quick trip to a supermarket we spent the rest of the day relaxing. My foot was aching by late afternoon, and my big toe and three middle toes felt numb, but the next day, I was active and realised I was doing things much earlier this time around and perhaps becoming complacent, but by 9 pm, I was in severe pain, so I went to bed.

The pain just intensified, and I had to give in and take some pain medication and was relieved that the tablets relaxed me enough to go to sleep. Intense pain in the early hours at Day 25 with a return of nausea and dizziness. Maybe my body was telling me I'd done too much? The wound was healing, and the scabs had peeled off. Back at home now after a wonderful weekend break.

Day 27 - I managed a quick visit to the supermarket – my dad pushed the trolley. I felt that I was getting back into a normal routine with regard to cooking meals and doing household chores.

My foot started to look better by day 30; although the scabs had peeled off the foot felt heavy after standing for too long and with some aching underneath. Daily chores increased and a return to my hobby of decorating cakes using an adjustable bar stool to keep the weight off my foot. There's only just over an inch of scab left on my foot. The scar line looked as if it would be as neat as the right foot now that more scab had peeled off.

My big toe and three of my middle toes still felt odd and numb. The area around the scar line felt incredibly sensitive and tender to the touch. However, my foot was feeling much sturdier and stronger. I looked forward to life without an Aircast boot.

Rose: Day 13 - after the nurse had cleaned the wound it looked much better. The blood blisters had started to dry up. I was given a small supply of dressings to change every couple of days, but the idea was to let the air get to the wound as much as possible. Wearing my Aircast boot meant I could walk without the aid of a crutch; I must admit that I found using two crutches at the same time didn't work for me as my balance was all over the place. At home, I made my way upstairs, this time on my feet, giving my bottom a well-deserved rest. The toe joint still felt stiff, but physiotherapy would help tremendously, as I recall from my past experience with the other foot. Having lost the encumbrance of the bandage I smothered my foot with moisturiser on the dry flaky skin. My foot started to look normal again.

Days 15–17- leaving the dressing off eased the soreness. The wound appeared nice and dry, without weeping, while the smaller scabs disappeared. The foot had a better wash in the bath this morning, being very gentle and I rested after last night but was back on my feet for probably a couple of hours, so I needed my Aircast boot. By the time I sat down after lunch, my foot was a little more swollen than normal, so I sat with the ice pack on, and after a couple of hours, the swelling went down; but the wound scabbing flaked off in little bits, but the larger bits stuck firmly without signs of stitch ends. The cream worked miracles and as it dried the wrinkly skin disappeared.

The wound on my other foot had taken longer to heal and required quite a few visits to the nurse to be dressed. I left the dressing off and replaced it with a light cotton sock.

After time spent downstairs, sitting, with my foot elevated, interspersed with washing and later cooking dinner, it was back to 'foot up' and ice in the evening.

The shooting pains came and went but on the whole were not giving me too much discomfort. The foot let me know when I'd done enough in the form of a 'burning' sensation, which disappeared after icing and elevation. The instep of my foot started to ache, so remembering my last physiotherapy session, I started rolling a tennis ball under the instep while seated to work and free the muscle up.

Day 20 - Soreness and throbbing eased off once I got out of bed. The remaining blood blister scab came off this morning, so my foot looks 'prettier'. The foot felt better than yesterday, with less throbbing, swelling, and redness upon waking. I hobbled around the supermarket in my Aircast boot before my appointment and had a severe 'telling off' and was sent for an X-ray, so I learned my lesson. Luckily, there wasn't any damage done—only to my pride.

A three-week milestone had now been reached, and I attended physiotherapy after using a taxi to the hospital. I was now managing without crutches. My physiotherapist was satisfied, and she proceeded to waggle my toes without causing me any discomfort at all. I felt really proud of myself and informed her how I had worked hard to keep the foot elevated for the past three weeks and that it had paid off. It would be nice to get into proper shoes for Christmas, although I wear flats most of the time so that wouldn't be any hardship. I was given a compression bandage to aid the swelling and returned home and sat with the foot up for an hour before ironing four shirts.

The compression bandage worked wonders for the swelling, and icing continued at least a couple of times a day. The time spent on my feet extended, but I had to elevate the limb after a couple of hours. Most of the scabbing has come off, leaving only the largest one. The shooting pains come and go, but they last only for a few seconds when they do come.

I continued my exercises as instructed and the tennis ball worked wonders on the muscles in my instep, which were feeling almost back to normal.

I knew I had overdone it again at day 27. My foot was swollen and inflamed despite regular icing but felt a lot better as I had lost the largest scab. Rest with elevation certainly helps and the swelling has reduced over the past two days. I'm walking around the house with a slipper and have reduced using the Aircast boot, which made my hip ache with a lop-sided gait. I wore it to go outside occasionally. Massage continued directly onto the scar. I'm now into my fifth week since surgery and hopefully when I see the physiotherapist next week the Aircast boot can be left off entirely. The shooting pains are less and less – all in all, everything is going nicely.

~ Rose's diary ended here ~

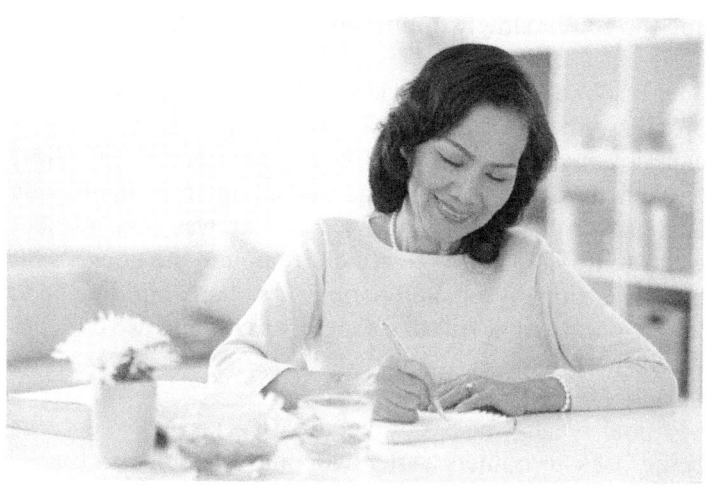

DAY 30+

Florinda: Walking around the house unaided has been without concern. I continued to use the Aircast boot and one crutch when going out, out of concern that someone would tread on my operated foot. I attempted to wear trainers, but these made my toe feel like it was being forced into an unnatural position. New trainers were purchased to accommodate my swollen foot. I felt stir crazy unable to go out when I wanted to but I have been fortunate to have friends who picked me up and took me out to help with this 'cabin fever'. This did not stop the frustration of being unable to get out when I wanted to drive myself. Unfortunately, I had an accident and tripped up a disabled ramped kerb. My operated toe took the brunt and was immediately painful. The foot swelled to the point where I could not put my shoe back on later that afternoon. The pain is more severe now than after surgery, with frequent sharp shooting pains and a constant throb. The swelling persisted and the colour slowly diminished.

Jackie: Week 5 - My physiotherapist was pleased with my progress. She got me to stand with both feet flat to the floor and flex my toes as far as I could, and there was a little movement in my big toe. I had to continue with the flexing exercises and to massage my foot but was able to start wearing my trainers (with crutches) around the house. This meant starting off for short periods, gradually building up to longer periods, but still to wear the Aircast and use crutches when I went out.

My goal when I next saw her two weeks later would be being back in trainers. After shopping I decided to try my trainers on and was quite shocked as they were very difficult to get on my left foot (despite being a larger size); it must be more swollen than I thought.

I walked around and left them on for about an hour, when my foot started to hurt so that was enough for today, but I was pleased with my progress. I used the trainers where I could, but had to fall back on the Aircast, as much as I did not like using it. I slowly built the trainers for up to four hours, used paracetamol where needed for any sharp shooting pain, and massaged the skin with cream. The numbness in the toes continued, but I saw a light at the end of the tunnel and a return to normal.

Week 6 - Things had progressed well but slowly, and I was back in my normal ankle boots while walking around the supermarket supported by the trolley. Bizarrely, my right foot (earlier surgery) was actually hurting far more than my left, and this continued for the rest of the week. The physio was impressed by my progress and how well I was walking. She got me to do some balancing exercises on high-density foam. I struggled at first, and the pain in my right foot didn't help, but I was recommended to continue at home to strengthen my core. For the pain in my right foot, the physiotherapist applied some felt underneath my foot (just before the ball of my foot) – I thought it was worth a try as I was feeling quite disappointed that my right foot now seemed to be holding me back. When I put my trainers back on I couldn't believe the difference – it seemed to give me support and the pain disappeared. The physiotherapist then discharged me.

The consultant arranged to see me in just over two months.I carried out the balancing as instructed and used my pad. Life started to return to normal although I hadn't driven, mainly because of the right foot pain. I hit 10,000 steps and walked 2.5 miles round trip into town twice this week. The Aircast boot was no longer required at Week 7 and the pain in both feet was minimal with the use of felt on the right foot.

There was some residual swelling in my left foot and the wound area was still tender to touch. Both feet appear stiff and tender when getting out of bed in the morning and walking downstairs.

Driving

Driving for short distances at week 8 caused my foot to ache when I got home. I certainly wouldn't have felt happy driving a long distance, but I did manage several short journeys during the week. It was busy due to Christmas and my feet ached as I had probably done too much. Achieving rest was not easy with such a busy family life. The left foot wound was still tender, and the foot was swollen. Sudden, sharp, needle-like pains occasionally arose through the toes, although they still felt numb and uncomfortable.

I had to cope with snow at week 10, but continued wearing the felt pads on both feet and reverted to a pair of very old, worn-out zip-down boots because, unfortunately, the new ones, which appeared to be comfortable, turned out to be far from snug. After a few days, I felt better in my old tatty boots. As snow arrived, I dreaded walking out in it, worrying about the cold on my feet or whether I would even fit into my wellies, but I managed to get them straight on. Walking was a challenge and I slipped several times but managed to save myself. During the evening I started to get very sharp pains in my left foot, which lasted for several hours. Paracetamol and ibuprofen eased the pain for a couple of days. The left foot swelled by night time and I had a general ache around my ankle.

More setbacks arose in weeks 12–14, after the Christmas preparations were well underway. I had ordered my festive food shop online as the thought of pushing a heavy trolley around a busy supermarket filled me with fear.

Whilst happily unpacking my goodies, the worst thing happened – a full two-litre bottle of lemonade fell out of the fridge and landed on my left big toe. The pain was intense, and I actually screamed and was reduced to tears. I was dreading the damage I may have done. I lay on the sofa, took a paracetamol and had a cup of tea to calm me down. I rested for an hour, and luckily, the pain subsided, and I was able to walk as normal. The next day, some bruising appeared, but it could have been so much worse. I think I had a very lucky escape.

On Christmas Eve we walked to a local restaurant with friends. I put on a pair of new boots as my comfy ones were just too scruffy to wear – bad decision! It set the pain off in my other foot. Christmas Day arrived, and I cooked dinner for ten people with help but by the afternoon my feet were throbbing and were incredibly uncomfortable – they needed much more rest than they'd been allowed. Boxing Day allowed me to rest. There was no let up for the rest of the week as it was my son's birthday, and a trip a film studio meant a whole day's walking.

Week 22 - I had my final post-operative checkup for my left foot, which was fine, but had to admit the problems with the right foot. A corticosteroid injection helped. The left foot caused no problems – the toes were still numb with achy stiffness when getting out of bed and walking downstairs in mornings, but this eased completely after a few minutes. The wound area was still tender to touch.

Jackie recorded her final diary entry six months after the surgery on her left foot, which was twelve months after her operation on her right foot.

Besides a dull ache at the end of hectic days and some discomfort after driving, I am certainly without the pain those awful bunions gave me.

As far as shoes go, I am still wearing flat boots, trainers or flat sandals. I have tried a slight heel but can't tolerate it for too long. It certainly hasn't been easy. Would I do it again, knowing what I know now? Yes, I would, but for me personally, it's been a difficult journey, though it's one worth taking. I would say that my right foot has fully recovered, but it has taken 12 months. Other than the numbness in the left foot, I am virtually pain-free. I can walk the dogs again and walk at a normal pace. I feel life has returned to normal.

§

Jackie's diary lasted the longest and had the greatest detail associated with some distinctive problems. Rose remained in touch for six months later and returned her follow-up questionnaire. Florinda was lost to follow up. A glossary of operative problems is provided later in part IV and covers some of the issues described in the diaries. From a clinician's view, it is useful to see the effects of our work and how patients manage, some better than others. Many of the descriptions provided are not presented in common information sheets for a good reason—everyone responds differently.

The cryotherapy jacket - reduces swelling and pain (Fig.4.4). The ice barrel is not shown but when filled with ice and cold water can cool effectively for around five hours

The Limbo Cover - This is not the only system on the market (Fig.4.6). Plastic bags can leak and lead to wet dressings, affecting wound healing. Purpose-designed covers are reinforced. The use of a waterproof chair provides balance when showering. Plastic collapsable chairs are available from the usual online suppliers.

Revision Surgeries

Revision means one of two things: the operation or procedure to fix your bunion did not go as planned, or the deformity recurred. One of our most common queries is whether the operation stiffened the toe without intention. In other cases, the dressings were removed, and the patient found that the toe had not corrected sufficiently. We reveal some behind-the-scenes evidence for why surgery may not always work without implying any sense of negligence.

Part of the reason might be that the surgery, while performed adequately, was not the right surgery for the extent of the high angle. In other cases, the sesamoid bones (recall these from Part I & II) failed to realign (Fig.4.7). Some surgeons will remove the outer sesamoid to remove the tension that causes recurrence.

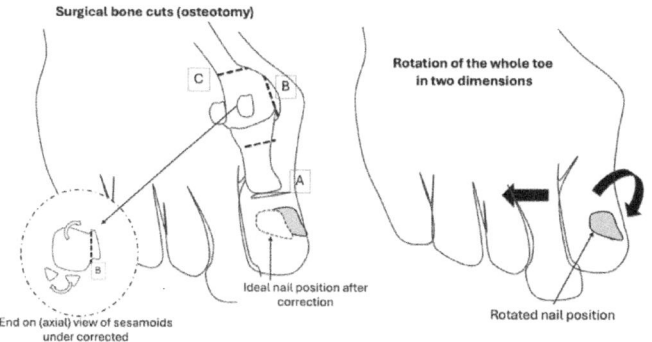

Fig.4.7. The toe deformity is challenging and can exist in more than one-dimensional plane once the toe rotates changing the nail position.

The other reason for the failure to correct may be a failure to appreciate that the toe is not deviated in one direction but two[53]. The left-hand image in Fig. 4.7. shows three potential operative sites to correct the toe position marked by dotted lines.

A—involves altering the angle in the proximal phalanx to aid better tendon pull.

B- removes sufficient bunion bump as an exostectomy. We have learned that too much bone removed causes additional problems.

C- forms the central part of the correction (See part II, Fig 3.5) which usually changes the metatarsal alignment with the sesamoids.

The smaller image in Fig. 4.7 —bottom left, illustrates the rotation effect. If surgery fails to make an adequate alignment with the osteotomy, recurrence can arise. Research is not easy to undertake as deformities come in different guises. One reason for fusing the toe joint is to reduce the risk of recurrence, and some surgeons still favour this approach.

The justification for destroying a joint, removing the integral cartilage, becomes a decision about long-term assurances against recurrence versus hobbled to limited footwear choice. The next cases reveal revision decisions and their outcomes.

---

[53] Dayton, P, Feilmeier, M, Kauwe,M, Hirschi,J. Relationship of frontal plane rotation of first metatarsal to proximal articular set angle and hallux alignment in patients undergoing tarsometatarsal arthrodesis for hallux abducto valgus: A case series and critical review of the literature. J.Foot & Ankle Surg. 52(2013)348-354

How long does bunion surgery last? A Twenty-Eight Year Follow-Up

Revision Surgery

While many published articles cite cases followed from one to five years this is probably insufficient to assess the longevity of correction. While foot surgeons try to select the best procedure and maintain a healthy joint, deformities can reoccur. Identifying an absolute cause is not easy, as scientific controls are complicated, given many variations called confounding factors.

We do know that surgery on young feet has a high chance of further deformity and is best left until later in life. In this next case study (2024—*edited*), a respondent wrote.

Patient – J - My hallux valgus was operated on at thirty-five. A wedge was removed from the first metatarsal, and the big toe had a pin insertion (Fig.4.8), marked as screw fixation. The surgery was very successful, both in terms of aesthetics and in resolving foot pain. I was able to get back to work as a pharmacist on my feet all day. Unfortunately, twenty-eight years on, I can see no alternative but to have a further procedure, as the condition has gradually reoccurred - and to an even greater extent now, with the big toe crossing over the second toe. This will undoubtedly cause balance problems as the big toe is not properly in contact with the floor, not to mention my embarrassment over the appearance of my foot and difficulty with footwear.

Aside from the post-operative discomfort and downtime and wanting to avoid a general anaesthetic, I also have concerns about finding a surgeon/hospital as my late Mum had a hallux valgus operated on by a surgeon at X Hospital, with a completely unsuccessful outcome.

As an expert in the field, I would like to know if you could advise me on how best to proceed. Would you have any pointers on the optimum technique/procedure to correct this (including any information on 'minimally invasive' procedures?)? Certainly, any knowledge of suitably experienced surgeons would be greatly appreciated. I only wish you were still operating!

Response:

Twenty-eight years is typically around the active lifespan of a surgeon[54]. Consult a dedicated foot surgeon, either a Fellow of the Royal College of Surgeons (FRCS) or from the Royal College of Podiatry (FRCPodS).

The base wedge osteotomy does cause a small amount of shortening (Fig.4.8.), so your most reliable, longer-term solution is to consider a joint fusion (arthrodesis).

The arthrodesis procedure stiffens the toe and sets for a specific heel height. Arthrodesis is regarded as the gold standard for revision work. The recurrence is unlikely and should last until the end of life, but most of us do not perform this as a first-line surgery as younger people prefer to opt for toe movement.

Select surgeons whose primary practice is foot surgery. Dedicated orthopaedic and podiatric surgeons are good at what they do, but experience in revision surgery is essential.

---

[54] This case was author DRT.

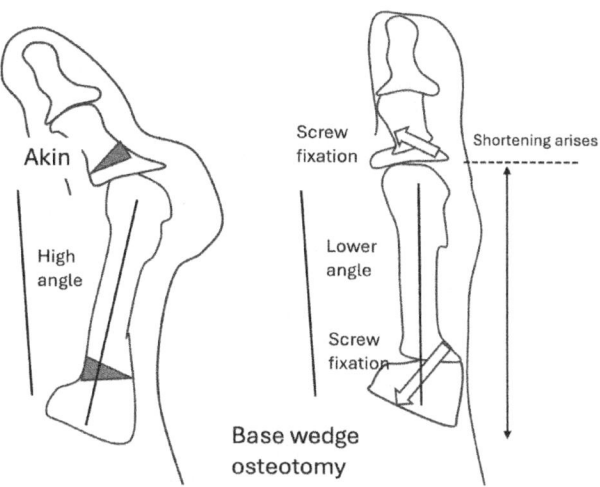

Fig.4.8.The base wedge osteotomy is favoured less as a first-line treatment. It is useful for large deformity angles but should be avoided if the first metatarsal bone length is initially short. The bone shortens in this procedure and allows good joint movement, but it can take up to a year or more to achieve this.

Patient J: My initial instinct is that it seems counter-intuitive to fuse a joint with no current stiffness or pain, and if the toe ends above the floor, it may not improve the balance issues. However, it makes sense that it would prevent the reoccurrence of the hallux valgus. I would like to hear your thoughts on minimally invasive surgery, if it is relevant to my situation.

Response: Revision surgery comes with heightened risks of failure and complications. The shortening of the bone is the most relevant. Long-term studies on bunion surgery need to meet scientific standards; a 30-year follow-up is unavailable. Revision surgery after several years after primary surgery can be successful.

Fusion is a safer bet than most alternatives and offers better longevity. Third surgeries seldom come without loss of function. More surgery involves deeper tissue scarring, and even then, a joint-sparing operation could lead to limited joint movement. Minimal incisional surgery (MIS) appeals to many for obvious reasons, but the follow-up is not as well presented as other surgeries and is limited to specific criteria. MIS is available and has advantages. New screw systems allow surgical placement through keyholes under X-ray-guided control.

Do not overburden the second surgeon with annoyance or disappointment with the first surgery. You cannot expect the second person to react in the way you wish they would respond to a colleague. You'll find that medicine is inevitably protective and cautious where everyone feels under scrutiny, perhaps more so today than ever before, with a high level of litigation. Avoid making statements advising on litigation or making any statement that claims negligence against the first surgeon.

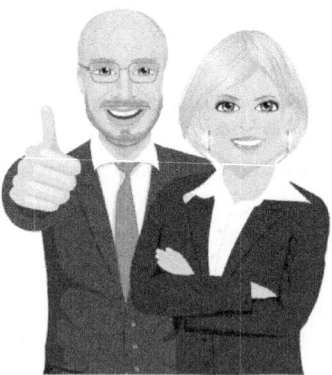

Fig.4.9 While surgery has been a male domain in the podiatric and orthopaedic fields, more women have taken up consultant posts in both these fields than previously.

Deciding who to seek assistance remains a post code lottery. For those prepared to travel, services offering an expedient appointment can be found.

Orthopaedic Surgeon Versus Podiatric Surgeon?

We don't believe it matters which surgeon you go to, but that person should be experienced and dedicated to the foot alone.

Some podiatric specialists undertake surgery work with orthopaedic teams.

Foot surgery is a highly specialised and risky area of the body. Not all surgeons have the breadth of surgical experience for complex revision surgery.

Rachel's Double Toe Surgery - Her Case Story 2012-2014

Rachel worked in a pharmacy department. She was forty-seven and had stiff toe joint pain. Rachel kept a log and stayed in touch for six months between 2017-18. We pick up her story in 2021 after four years.

Rachel had a painful bunion on each foot. She had the right foot managed first in 2012 and received an implant (*plastic hinged joint*). Her left foot had an osteotomy (bone cut procedure) in 2014. The right foot had more cartilage damage than the left foot.

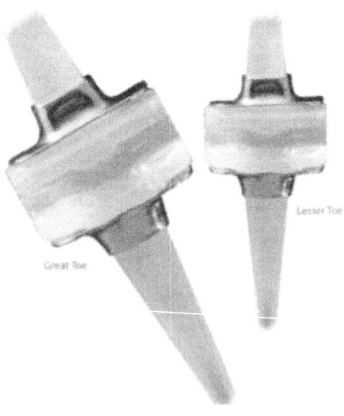

Fig. 4.10. Silastic (silicone implants to replace damaged joints)

CLINICIAN COMMENT

It is usual to try to maintain healthy cartilage using an osteotomy. By 2017, Rachel was not doing so well, and it was clear that a new approach was required. As her right foot did so well, she elected to have a revision surgery using the silastic implant. Some osteotomies fail. We don't have a figure on conversion from osteotomy to other surgery, but this might be estimated at 5%. Surgery is reserved for when all other treatment has failed, or the joint is irreversibly damaged. Surgical joint management involves the joint being removed entirely and either left with a gap or a spacer being introduced into the gap. In Rachel's case, the surgeon had to convert the osteotomy to a silastic prosthetic joint.

This is Rachel's diary —

The Day of Surgery

The operation went well as I knew what to expect; the best part was the anaesthetic; is it wrong that I find it so relaxing? No pain when I came around. I didn't feel the need for pain medication but took some before going to bed, even though the pain was very minimal. The anaesthetic block was still in place. I stayed at my parent's bungalow, so getting to the toilet was much easier than shuffling on my bum up the stairs. All in all, the first day and night were comfortable.

After Surgery

Day 1 - Foot still very numb, still no pain, but continued to take the pain medication just in case. I could see the bruising at the end of my toes, which is to be expected, I started to wiggle my toes and even wiggle the big toe a little. I am not too good at resting, so I helped my parents put the Christmas tree up. It was a stupid thing to do as the foot was very sore by mid-afternoon. I need to remember I only had the operation yesterday - so the foot is now resting and elevated. I was feeling a lot better by early evening. Another good night's sleep on pain medication.

Day 2 - It's an uncomfortable morning. It feels like the block has really worn off now. The foot feels stiff and sore. I'm trying to wiggle as much as I can. I don't know if I am supposed to be doing this, but it helps to loosen off. I had to take pain meds this morning, but all in all, it was a good day.

Day 3 - Pain is minimal; I wouldn't call it pain as such; it is more of a tingling sensation and slightly sore. Again, it felt very stiff and lumpy underneath, but from experience, I knew it would feel like this. I rested the foot as much as possible today, although I did get in the shower with the leg sleeve (Limbo cover) for the first time today. I can't say enough how wonderful it was to get under that water. I feel as though I haven't showered for weeks. The foot pulled a bit afterwards, but the pain meds kicked in quickly. I still have to heel walk, which isn't the easiest thing to do, I can't wait to get the air boot on tomorrow.

CLINICIAN COMMENT

Showers are not recommended too early because of the risk of falling. Appropriate rails and support are best. You can buy temporary handles to stick on tiles or glass to act as safety grips. A chair that can be used under the shower also helps with foot surgery. A specialised jacket is better than a plastic bag. Plastic bags can rip and also do not have a viable waterproof seal. All our patients were provided with ice (cryotherapy jackets) and plastic covers.

Day 4 - First appointment with the nurse today. I can't wait to get out of this blue (post-operative) shoe and get the air boot on. The nurse changed the dressing; I couldn't look – I wouldn't say I like the sight of blood, so when I saw it all over the bandage, it turned my stomach; needless to say, that was the worst bit. The wound was amazing, so clean and tidy. I had bruising to the toes, but such a neat job – wonderful consultant job yet again. I'm disappointed – I can't have the air boot on until my next appointment the following week as I still need to heel walk.

CLINICIAN COMMENT

The AircastTM boot is often called a walker cast (Fig.4.4). It is made from a heavy plastic two-piece shell with a hefty curved sole that allows the foot to rock forward safely, limiting discomfort. Large dressings must be reduced, as too much padding will cause pressure. Rachel describes her disappointment but once the Aircast is used she knows from past experience that her mobility will double.

Day 5 - I am back in my home today, so I am tackling the stairs, walking sideways up and coming down on my bum. My foot is slightly tender today, but nothing I cannot deal with. Again, having gone through this before, I think my brain knows what to expect. Had it been the first time, I might have been more uncomfortable. I am probably doing too much; the nurse did tell me off (a little) yesterday, and as she could see, I was trying to run before I could walk. There was lots of rest today, foot up, and Christmas movies. Evening – first time cooking for myself as I have been waited on hand and foot by my parents for the last few days. Cooking was okay, but standing washing up, my foot became tender. I elevated the foot on cushions for the evening, but no need for pain meds as I am not good at taking tablets so only take when I am in real bad pain. Had a great night's sleep in my own bed. The winter quilt was a bit heavy, so my foot poked out of the bed most of the night, but the cold actually felt good on it.

Day 6 - I had a good night's sleep and decided to try walking the dog with my parents today. Big mistake; I was only out for ½ an hour. My foot was so tight and sore afterward, and to top it all off, I stubbed my toe on a cabinet. It was nothing that pain meds couldn't sort out, but I need to realise my foot needs resting more. I felt very sore during the evening, and it felt lumpy underneath, but I still only felt a bit of discomfort.

Day 7 - I had a good night's sleep again with no pain. I am still finding the quilt a bit heavy on my foot. I could use one of those cages to hold the quilt off!! I did a bit of shopping at the supermarket today with my parents. I used crutches, so it's not too bad. However, walking around with my shoes on is giving me a backache. Perhaps I am being too cautious and not putting as much pressure on as I should, but I have been told to heel walk for the first seven days.

Day 8 - Not able to get out today so going a bit stir crazy. I can't wait to get the air boot on now so I can at least go up the garden with the dog. Missing my long walks with him, I must stop feeling impatient. I have been trying to bend my toe. It's so stiff and I have flinched a couple of times, maybe I should wait until I go to physiotherapy. Stood and did a bit of ironing. The toe are stiff and uncomfortable but not painful. I do feel it when I eventually put my feet up. It's like a fuzzy feeling through the whole of my foot, almost like when you have had really bad pins and needles. I want to bang my foot on the floor to get rid of it, but obviously I don't."

Six Months Later

The foot is fantastic, the best thing I did was go ahead and have the replacement joint, although I still get a certain amount of swelling, especially after a long walk, which I am now back up to speed with. I am walking the dog approximately 3–3.5 miles each day. If the weather is warm, it swells up more, but a bag of frozen peas for half an hour soon settles it down. My foot has gone down from a size 5 to a size 4.5, making it easier to buy shoes.

Four Years Follow Up

My foot is progressing well; I must admit it gives me pain at times, mainly through the Winter months when my foot is cold. I have at times struggled to walk as it swelled up so much so that a few months ago, I was going to contact the surgeon to get advice on who to see as I felt it might need x-raying. Alongside the pain, it does cause me to have problems with my lower back as I am probably not walking on the foot at all times due to the pain; it can actually wake me up in the night with shooting pains, not very often but when it does it is very painful.

CLINICIAN COMMENT

Revision surgery can make the foot sensitive to cold. Nerves associated with scar tissue also seem less able to function and may be akin to dental nerve pain when those fillings are no longer working. Metalwork within the surgery, screws, plates, and anything that is not made by the body will conduct heat and cold differently. The solution is to add insulation to the shoes or socks. Keep the skin supple at all times, and avoid hot water bottles. The technique of massage is aided by cream or oils. Medication can reduce shooting pains. Always look to a healthy diet with fresh vegetables and vitamins, especially oily fish. Maintain exercise as much as possible to work the leg and foot muscles. Back pain arises because the foot/feet are imbalanced. This can be solved by having your gait analysed by a podiatrist and using fitted orthoses.

Tom's Story - When Things Are Not Quite Right?

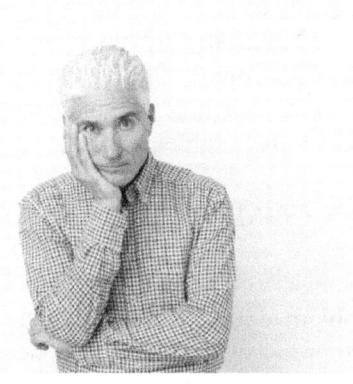

Tom was 80 at the time of surgery and first saw his surgeon for a trigger finger but complained about his big toe as well after being asked if there were any other problems. He ended up talking about his left big toe, which became the narrative for the consulting session. Many parts are attributed to Tom's voice -

'I took my shoe off,' Tom said.

Surgeon —'Ah, classic hallux rigidus. I'll tell you what. I'll do that at the same time as I do your trigger finger. I could fuse it, but it'd be much better to have a replacement silastic joint. It'll give you more movement, and that's what I recommend.'

I didn't think anything at all but it was beautifully casual. You walked yourself into the operating theatre and you climbed up onto the bed, before the anaesthetist got to work.

Anyway, it was very successful, and it was great for about twelve years and then began to hurt.

Twelve Year Follow Up

For the last couple of years, I couldn't walk properly. I had to walk on my heel on the outside of my foot to protect the toe. After playing a round of golf, it hurt like hell, about the fifteenth and sixteenth holes, and then it got to the stage where I couldn't play eighteen holes.

CLINICIAN COMMENT

Rachel's case was the reverse of Tom's story. The most common problem with silastic implants is when the hinge tears and compresses, losing any functional value. The use of a metal washer (grommet) helps minimise this. The manufacturer advises a year life-span. We have seen these last 7-20 years. They can be replaced with a second spacer. Leaving the implant to age 55-60 means the implant does less work as activity reduces. Spacers and joints, therefore, have a limited lifespan. Because many foot surgeons are unhappy with the unpredictability of prosthetic implants, they offer a stiffening procedure.

Tom sought a second consultation with a different surgeon. Revision surgeries are not always easy.

He said, "This is a tricky procedure because I'm going to have to do a bone graft, and I'm also going to have to do a skin graft because there won't be enough skin." he proposed lengthening the toe as it had shortened.

Tom asked, "Why can't you just amputate the toe?" The surgeon did not recommend this.

CLINICIAN COMMENT - amputations

Amputations should only be undertaken when all other methods cannot be performed. The toe is important in pushing off from the foot during walking (Fig.1.10), and weight distribution across the ball of the foot is better engineered if the toe is present.

Overwhelming bone infection from poor healing was required in one older patient with good results and return to normal function, but such cases are rare. Her ulcer had failed to heal for several years, and she had marked rheumatoid arthritis.

Another year went by, and it got more painful, and I went back to the GP, and he sent me to a different man."

The surgeon reiterated to Tom that it was a tricky procedure and that bone and skin grafts would be needed.

Third Opinion

I sought a third opinion. Now the consultation was slightly different. The later surgeon said to me, 'I don't think it's necessary to lengthen the toes. I don't have to do a skin graft, and I'm fairly confident you will be pleased with the outcome.' He explained everything that could go wrong. Curiously, the surgeon said, 'I've never had an operation myself, and I never want one because I know what can go wrong.'

There is no clear guide on seeking multiple opinions. The danger remains in moving from one to another in order to hear the words that best fit one's desire. The reader must make their own decision in the case of Tom.

CLINICIAN COMMENT

Patients will recall minor details within conversations, but engaging with multiple consultations can be equally confusing as helpful. It is perfectly reasonable to seek another opinion, and Tom is looking for a) the best outcome and b) surgery that has the lowest risk and interference with his life. Revision surgery is a specialty in its right and so no patient wants to be made worse.

Planned Surgery Goes Ahead

After getting multiple opinions, his surgery included a bone graft taken from the hip.

Up until probably two weeks ago, I regretted doing it very much because the surgeon impressed upon me how incredibly important it was to keep the foot elevated for 15 minutes out of every hour. I did find lying on my back with the foot up difficult to cope with.

Before I went, after I'd done some activity like trying to play golf or mowing the grass, the pain would be 7 out of 10, and it would last most of the night. It would keep me awake, and it would get swollen. After I had the operation, for the first two or three weeks, it was sort of 7 all the time. And then then it became about 5 of 10.

CLINICIAN COMMENT - **Bone lengthening and skin grafts**

Revision surgery is always riskier because scar tissue can increase. Scar tissue comprises fibrous *collagen* and tethers around nerves and blood vessels, ultimately sticking to cartilage and joint linings. Physiotherapy assists rebuild the movement after surgery. The toe can shrink in length, and so functionally, the toe fails to work as it once would. Building the missing gap with bone is important, and traditionally, this comes from the pelvis. The iliac crest offers the best quality bone and, as it comes from the patient, offering the best bonding. If the toe lengthens, the skin may become over-tight, and a skin supplement may be required. Generally this is not necessary unless the shortening of the toe was extensive and needs to be stretched.

Tom was followed up at six weeks with X-rays and advised to stay in his rigid shoe. A registrar explained his surgery and its complexity to Tom. Later, NS told Tom that the plastic had destroyed some of the bones.

Based on this, the surgeon said it would take a bit longer, which disappointed me. I needed more time and would be seen again in three months. I tried putting a shoe on and found I could get one on. And it began to feel better. The X-ray showed that the bone had knitted together satisfactorily. It was a big, big plate. The plate they put in covers the whole length of the wound. It's about four inches, I would say, and it had a lot of screws in it. I was amazed at how many screws it had. I think there were at least four on each side. There were about eight screws in the whole thing.

The surgeon was satisfied that everything had gone well and advised that Tom would not do any harm and could start doing normal things.

I played two nine holes, and the discomfort was a bit less than before I went to have it done. And right now, the pain is two or three out of ten. I'm aware of it, but it's not bad. I find that when I wake up in the morning, the pain is zero. When I wake up in the morning, there's a nice gap between all my toes, and at night time, when I go to bed – particularly if I've done something – it's swollen, and there's no gap between toes. I asked the guy when I saw him if that was anything to worry about.

Tom was informed that he had at least another nine months before he would get the full benefit.

It's nasty, and it feels as if the skin has been burnt. It's a bit like a shingles pain, but it tends to be only when you touch it. Most of the time, I'm unaware of it; it's just touching it.

CLINICIAN COMMENT

Most people judge success by the time it takes to recover and return to normal life. What is recovery? When is normal normal? Tom's gauge was returning to golf without pain. Massaging scars is an important consideration and can help desensitise wounds.

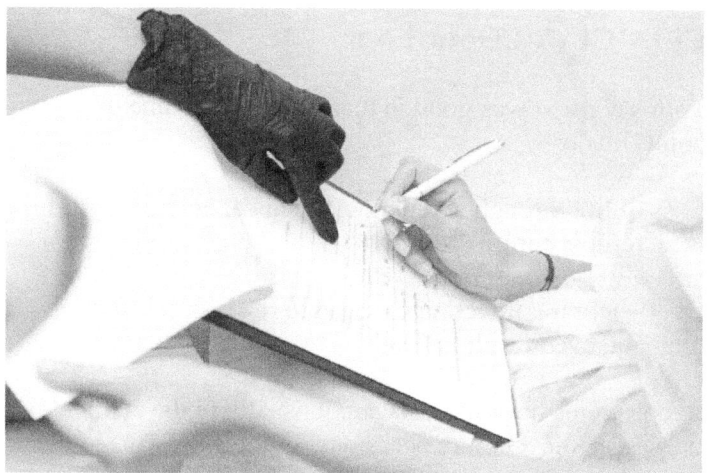

Consent

By 2010, consent in the UK had received much debate in the medical profession. Standards have improved from the preceding years. The patient allows the surgeon to undertake physical harm based on delivering benefits.

However, consent is where things can go wrong. It may not surprise the reader that this area of our work is the most hotly contested. Tom was asked when he gave consent.

> I was asked to sign a consent form in the clinic, which I did. He was very blunt and honest about everything that could go wrong. He told me about deep vein thrombosis and that I could die and if everything went terribly wrong I could get a lot of infection. I might lose my foot, he said. I didn't feel he was putting any pressure on me to do it. But he did give me confidence.

CLINICIAN COMMENT

Tom's consent was good in that he recalled some of the big points made:—

Loss of life through an unknown medical emergency. This is mercifully rare.

Overwhelming infection can lead to the loss of a foot or limb and even result in death.

Deep venous thrombosis is a clot usually in the calf and is fully treatable. On rare occasions, a clot can fly off to the lung (pulmonary thrombosis) and is life-threatening.

What is often not mentioned is numbness and nerve damage.

Overwhelming pain can be caused by a rare and unusual problem called complex regional pain syndrome. The risk can increase with multiple surgeries.

Slow healing is not uncommon after big toe surgery, although it may only affect a small portion of the wound. Scar tissue causes nerves to be bound down with some tenderness with a light touch.

Hardware removal due to movement or, breakage, or allergy can all cause symptoms.

Behind the Scenes

How had things gone for Tom?

Part of Tom's concerns has been that he had several surgeries without making a fuss.

- When armed with all the information, why did his hospital want to repeat tests when they had been done before?
- Why was he rejected and referred back to the general hospital when so close to surgery?
- Against these delays, why, when he was suffering, was he bounced back and forth with no action?

Tom illustrates the frustrations of disappointment at being cancelled and overwhelmed by the machinery of health service admission policy. He had been experiencing problems with revision toe surgery for several years. Initially, the outcome of his surgery was satisfactory after his original plastic joint was removed for an arthrodesis procedure (Fig.4.3).

Golf activity makes for a good assessment of foot health—problems with the arthrodesis procedure is fairly uncommon but then all surgical procedures have their weak spots.

Tom's second (revision) surgery had not gone that well. He started to notice a dark pigment in the skin of the left, operated foot and symptoms had not been relieved as he has expected. His expectations had been disappointing, and he gauged this by his ability at golf, now reduced by the number of holes to 50%. This story is about unexpected delays and frustrations.

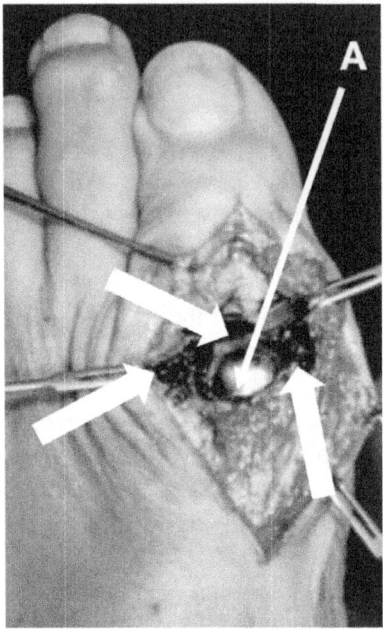

Fig.4.11. Metallosis around metal implants showing a metal joint. A – identifies the metal surface of the implant. The broad arrows represent the blackened tissue, similar in Tom's case when plates were used instead of a metal joint.

The author (DRT) met with Tom who opened a folder containing his notes, various results, and some ECG traces. Tom was asked if he had had any setbacks after his original revision in 2019. Until nine months after surgery Tom's toe was improving. Then it deteriorated.

> There is dark, purply-coloured skin under the skin. Pain is in my arch and on the outside of the ankle. I'm struggling to walk and regret having the surgery. I cannot wear some of my shoes, and the toe sticks up by 5-7cm.

CLINICIAN COMMENT

Common problems include movement of screws, fracture of a screw or loosening. He might have a break in the metal plate. The staining described can be associated with metallosis. Allergy to the metal is rarer. Metallosis is usually reported with implants containing metal and plastics. The figure (Courtesy Podiatry Institute 2017) shown is a combination which resulted from a toe implant rather than a plate (Vanore & O'Keefe).[55]

Metallosis has been seen in plates for toe joint arthrodesis and implant metal components. Owing to the thin skin, the colour can be alarming. Tom recalls no information about the findings at surgery.

Delays, Frustrations & Protocols

Tom was able to have surgery in a local private hospital, and after somewhat of a delay, largely around the post-COVID period of NHS chaos, he was all set for surgery. The use of the independent sector is far from new, and today, the NHS rely on the additional capacity for elective procedures—these are operations with low risk.

Tom is a fit-looking man. He knows he has slowed down, and the large garden he once cared for is now too much, so downsizing made sense. Now, he feels disappointment, perhaps more about the delays and setbacks.

---

[55] http://www.podiatryinstitute.com/pdfs/Update_2017/Chapter6_final.pdf —"Problematic" Implant or Complications of First metatarsophalangeal joint Implant Arthroplasty.

Relocating from a larger property also meant having to change doctors, although a letter to chase up delays finally resulted in surgery but not in the originally planned independent hospital. We looked at some of the background problems. On the surface it appeared his delays were partly beaurocratic confusion, COVID-19 and to a lesser extent, moving house. There were medical reasons for some of Tom's delays.

Health Issues

Tom takes a standard diet of heart medication, which is common to many men over the age of sixty. However, this generally is fine if all is stable, as the medication reduces the latent risks from further heart disease. Ensuring patient safety is paramount. After all, it is embarrassing to lose a patient on the operating table through poor assessment of a patient unsuited to surgery! There are two elements: *the anaesthetic and the surgical recovery.* Tom slips into the first of these two concerns.

Pre-admission

An experienced nurse will undertake a questionnaire and arrange blood tests and an ECG for specific categories of patients before admission. Tom's ECG threw up two problems—a previous myocardial infarction and a right-*sided nerve conduction* problem called a bundle block.

Myocardial infarction (MI)

The heart is essentially muscle and pumps with its own blood supply (coronary vessels). If these vessels are blocked, then part of the muscle can die off, which affects the contraction (squeezing pressure). Death of muscle due to blood supply depletion is called infarction.

In most cases, patients recover fully and with medical supervision. Sometimes, MI may not even produce symptoms and is picked up by a routine ECG trace.

Bundle Block

Right branch bundle block (RBBB) means the nerve conduction required to stimulate the heart squeeze is faulty so that part of the heart (ventricle) does not contract and allow the squeeze pressure to work as well. The reasons for RBBB are given below, but RBBB occurs more frequently in men than women. Here are some causes of RBBB.

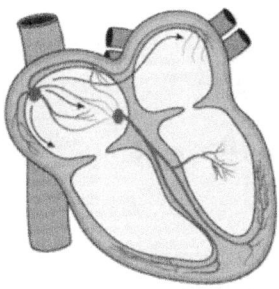

Fig.4.12. Shows nerves influencing the left and right side of the heart.

Cardiac Problems

Heart disease from high blood pressure
Chronic obstructive lung disease or COPD
A blood clot in the lung, otherwise known as a pulmonary embolism
Right-sided heart failure
Cardiomyopathy, which is a disease of the heart muscle
Idiopathic fibrosis or degeneration in the right bundle branch
Cardiac surgery
Myocarditis - inflammation of a membrane surrounding the heart
Aberrant ventricular conduction
Congenital heart disease
Coronary artery disease
Heart attack
Surgical procedures on the heart

As the right side is more intimately connected to the lungs receiving renewed oxygen, any defect can give rise to problems, especially under general anaesthetic (GA).

GA-based procedures introduce drugs that alter lung function, so breathing is assisted during an operation. Under conditions where someone has no medical problems, the risks are small. The reverse is true with medical problems, especially cardio-respiratory disease (heart-lung).

The Difference Between a UK Private Hospital & NHS General Hospital.

There can be no doubt that Tom's experience were hardly minor concerns from his perspective. Tom is a highly intelligent man who can process complex technical information. The healthcare professions can on many occasions provide digestible information but reliance on stock publications often removes the human element, and the surgeon resorts to information sheets to make up for the lack of explanation.

Tom contracted Covid at one point so an additional delay was likely. Still, he remained in the dark about being rejected as he reasonably deduced he had had surgery under general anaesthetic before without concern. The explanation above provided the core rationale and tended to be related to general anaesthetic based procedures. However, independent (private) hospitals do not have an intensive care bed or facility. The NHS run general hospitals are the only places where 24-hour staffing equipped to deal with emergency cases. Such facilities are unavailable in the independent sector who have to screen out high risk medical disease.

Specialised Intensive Care

Some independent hospitals have intensive care but this is based on strict protocols (rules) allowing care of the dying from cancer. Some high-staff-resourced care is undertaken, but not for unknown medical complications. Since the NHS decanted care to independent hospitals, rules were implemented to ensure that certain categories were screened and rejected if a potential risk was identified. Tom fell into this category but was not given a sufficient explanation.

The confusing feature is that private care (paid for by patients or insurers) can circumvent the NHS protocols, which appear at odds when defining risk. Curiously, Tom was offered follow-up tests at his expense despite him being an NHS referral.

The anomaly of private cases not following the same strict rules as the NHS referrals to those hospitals still exist. It comes down to the admissions (screening) nurse, the medical advisory committees and ultimately, the hospital manager, who can change the course of someone's admission. Most consultants will review any concerns raised, and admission will not proceed, particularly when the consultant anaesthetist is correctly involved. It is important to add most decisions are taken by others, not the surgeons involved with treatment.

Spinal blocks provided by anaesthetists and limb blocks, as performed by podiatrists, can avoid general anaesthetic, which immediately reduces the risk posed by the type of problem Tom had. A spinal anaesthetic was discussed but rejected by the anaesthetist, who had found Tom a poor candidate from previous experience.

After Revision Surgery

Tom's foot (when interviewed) was now eight + weeks after all the metalwork had been removed. The scar was fine and flat, and his foot, even in August when temperatures hit 28^{C}, was not swollen abnormally. The skin was not discoloured as it had once been. The toe was stiff and slightly shorter than the right foot's big toe. From a clinical point of view, all looked sound, and the procedure had achieved its aim – but not from Tom's viewpoint.

Risks From Surgery

One surgery is always best. The tissue is virgin except for any pathology found during the operation. The wound is sewn up (sutured), and this is when matters start to follow their own course. The material used can set off a reaction and increase inflammation as the body fights to absorb material designed to be left in.

The benefits must be weighed when we drift to a second or third surgery. *Could I be made worse? Should I stick with what I have?* The first surgery created scar tissue, and the virgin anatomy has now changed at the bone, joint and skin level.

The nerves – which are critical, can change the messaging service to the brain. Numbness is the best and most common example. However, some nerves are designed to recall pressure, some heat and cold, and others pain. In other words, there are specialist nerves. Nerves interact with chemicals, and these chemicals are produced by the body within the surgical site associated with inflammation.

Adapting After Surgery

After foot surgery, we alter our way of walking, which often is not always beneficial. Walking differently causes pain, and revision surgery takes longer to recover. As we age, we heal more slowly than when we were young. When Tom discussed the potential for revision surgery not always working, he accepted this. However, most patients retain positive hope and an optimistic outlook.

Patient Correspondence

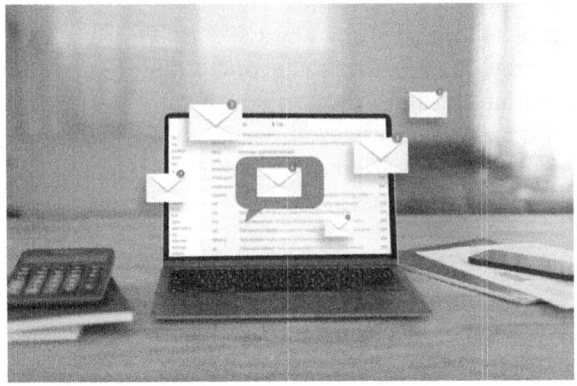

We have selected a range of authentic email queries concerning bunion surgery[56]. This represents a female audience from the UK and USA— no question is too simple or ridiculous.

All correspondents have provided permission and sent in photos to be used for educational purposes through the website consultingfootpain.co.uk. All family names, locations, and hospital names have been removed. Queries range from swelling, pain, healing, short toes after surgery, and types of operation.

---

[56] ConsultingFootPain (CFP) was established in 2014 as an information resource for consultations and contained clinical information for patients. In 2018 the website broadened its remit and now receives many thousands of hits each week and queries about different clinical matters.

Javell: Hi, I'm 6 weeks post-metatarsal osteotomy and Akin osteotomy lateral release and excision of Morton neuroma removal between 3/4 toe, all on the right foot. Healing well, I still can't fully weight bear barefoot. The toes are still stiff, and swelling occurs when standing for too long. I'm wearing shoes outside but barefoot indoors. However, my big toe and 2nd toe seem to have quite a gap. Will this eventually close? If so, when? Also, is there anything I can purchase to help the gap close any sooner

CFP: Hi Javell – I can only offer a general comment as I don't know all your details. The surgeries combined are fairly intensive and swelling can be sustained for 12-16 weeks so you have some way to go. The gap usually reduces with the swelling and walking, but I expect you to be loading the foot at six weeks as part of rehabilitation. The time that the foot will take weight can be slow. In 2-5% of cases, correction of the first toe can arise and leave a permanent gap. After many years operating, we have only corrected a few cases, but that decision should only be made later.

Kate: I had bunions removed on both feet 14 months ago. The left went great, the right, which was bigger, was good, and the swelling was going down, then stopped. Something was sticking in bottom of foot identified as sesamoid bone. This was shaved which stopped the pain but swelling remained the same as before shaving. Doc said swelling would go down but at six weeks it hasn't changed. I think it's still the same swelling from bunion surgery not the shaving.

How do I find out what is causing this. It gets sore when pressed during exercising, walking extended periods. There is no infected wound. Thanks.

CFP: Thanks, Kate, for your query. If the left foot deformity was larger, did you have the same operation performed? Sesamoid pain can be tricky; additional swelling may be related to shaving the bone and prolonged subsequent recovery. However, something sticking in your foot might require a clinical assessment with an X-ray. Swelling recovery is never easy to predict, and I feel extending this to at least four months might be sensible so you have less worry. Often two feet do not follow the same progress.

I need to know more about the type of procedure performed and what internal metalwork was used. I cannot be more specific at this time.

Debbie - Part I

Debbie: I had bunion and hammer toe (Fig.4.13) surgery eleven weeks ago. After severe pain in my foot and ankle after four weeks (& first wearing a trainer) an X-ray showed arthritis in the foot and ankle. Am now having physio & my surgeon says everything looks good, but it will be a slow recovery. I've been trying to walk daily – up to 1.5 or 2 miles, which I can manage but have pain afterwards. When I ask how far I should walk I just get told 'as far as you feel able'. Is this too much too soon? My husband and I used to walk miles, so I think I'm pushing myself to get back to this level quickly. Anyone else had this issue? Thanks

CFP: Debbie, there is no absolute right period before full activity. Patients may require 12-16 weeks for most resolution to occur and allow activity, including walking and dancing and playing sports. Some people do better earlier, and some take six months. The difference is the type of surgery (extent), age, your organic make-up, healing power, attitude, weight and determination. The advice from your surgeon is broadly correct. We appreciate your feelings of frustration, of course, not least because your husband is free to walk and wants you back. Please don't be too hard on yourself; you are nearly there but do build up with positive and yet realistic expectations.

Debbie: Thank you so much for your reply which has really reassured me. I think I have been putting too much pressure on myself to be honest. I need to listen to my body (which is what I would say to someone else as I am a nurse!) I've backed off walking for two days and had my first swim yesterday, which was great as it's one of my favourite activities. I also sat in the jacuzzi for five minutes & the heat really seemed to help. My mood really lifted too. I think you're right. Positive but realistic expectations! Thanks so much again. Your support has really helped me.

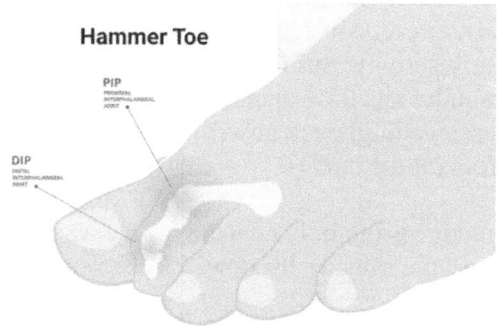

Fig. 4.13.

Debbie - Part II

A delay between messaging and Debbie came back again with more queries—five weeks on.

Debbie: Hi, Sorry to trouble you, but I've been reading the information on the CFP website and found it very informative. I hope you don't mind me asking, but I've undergone bunion surgery and would like to know if pain should still be an issue five weeks in. I have been elevating my foot as much as I can, though, trying to work the foot while in post-op shoes. All was well at my two-week post-op appointment, and I'm due to review my appointment. The wound still feels very tight and still, pain daily (though able to sleep with Co-codamol[57] if needed), and dressings would have a tiny smear of pink when changing them, but no discharge. I would appreciate your opinion on this—many thanks.

CFP: This is the most common question asked, and recovery is based on many different criteria, so we all vary in how we respond after surgery.The Scarf osteotomy is one of the top choice by foot surgeons in the UK, (*although not sure about the USA*) because it allows rapid recovery and is very stable. Are you UK based? While I encourage early activity, this has to be tempered by realistic limits and includes swelling management. A tight sensation would suggest swelling; even now, you will need to elevate and ice the foot (at the ankle).

Your pink smudge is our only concern, as the wound should have healed on the outside by now. Please send a quality image.

---

[57] Cocodamol is a prescription medicine used in the UK and a codeine based paracetamol painkiller. It is powerful and can produce side effects. USA acetaminophen with codeine.

Consider including a close-up and a picture of both feet for comparison. Please state your age and, if you have returned to work, and your occupation. Pain, ideally if present, should not arise at night or rest, but maybe uncomfortable on walking or standing too much and shouldn't need co-codamol at five weeks. Paracetamol should deal with the problem. There are exceptions, and those may exist around poor pain tolerance.

Reduce your activity, rest regularly with your foot up and if within 48 hours this does not improve and reduce the tightness, try bringing the appointment closer. Were you were treated under the NHS or Independent sector, as protocols may vary.

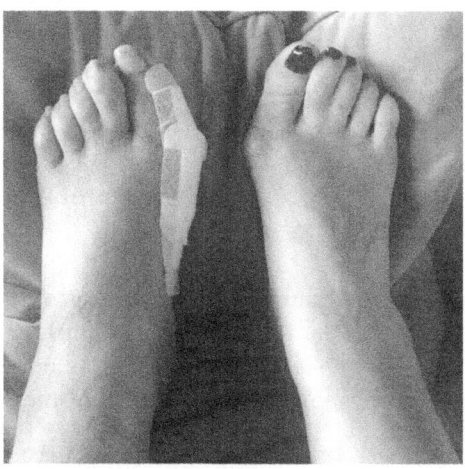

Fig.4.14. Debbie's foot after surgery. The result would have been disappointing, as the hallux is still very much impinging on the second toe. CFP did not make such a comment, but Debbie would require revision surgery.

Debbie: Thank you for your reply. I am 60 and have not yet returned to work.

I am a Learning Support Assistant in primary education, so the nature of my work includes being in a busy classroom of thirty children on a daily basis. I will continue with elevation and ice on the foot. Can I ask if dressing should still be used or best left to the air while at home. The tightness is across the top of the foot and the wound site, and there is always some degree of discomfort that stops me from placing the foot fully down when getting about.

CFP: Thanks, Debbie, for the pictures. The swelling is within normal limits. The wound has not quite healed, and the swelling is causing a little strain on the wound hence the leakage. It is not serious. There should be no untoward concerns as long as you don't smoke. You should not return to a classroom for a few more weeks as children are renowned for treading on feet accidentally. We routinely sign my teachers and TAs off for three months as standard to stop classroom pressures. Put bluntly; you are a health and safety risk until the wound is healed and swelling under more control. Try leaving the dressing off and wearing soft shoes or none around the house. The aim is to allow the wound to heal without too much covering.

Start with light creaming around the wound rather than in open areas. Don't bathe the foot for too long as this opens the skin.The aim is to rub hand cream around the edges of the wound, pushing down and back toward the ankle with gentle strokes. Build the pressure as you get used to the sensation. Timewise, do this for 30-90 seconds, then gradually up to three minutes if you can after a week+. Carry on with this until there is no scar tenderness. Once the wound has healed, that is, the edges are not raised, then massage the cream over the surgical incision, and with circling motions with the tips of the fingers, press until you cannot tolerate the discomfort. The type of cream does not matter as long as it is not greasy.

Hand or foot cream - the physical action, not the product, will densify the skin and make it better three times daily if you can. If the pain calms and you can cope with paracetamol, wait until you see your consultant next. Write any questions down to ensure you have an answer. Ask if there is any information they can give you, as this is standard practice for all surgeries.

Patients are not expected to guess; if you were seen after having had a general anaesthetic, chances you won't remember. Ask if you can have some physiotherapy, but don't be surprised if they say it isn't required, but it can help with walking re-education, restore confidence, and provide emotional support.

Debbie: I will continue with elevation and ice on the foot. Can I ask if dressing should still be used or best left to the air while at home. The tightness is across the top of the foot and the wound site, and there is always some degree of discomfort which stops me from trying to place the foot fully down when getting about. I will let you know how things go, thank you. I'm wondering if bathing the foot in sea water is a good idea yet or not as it isn't fully healed?

CFP: As long as the water is clean rather than polluted.

Debbie: I'm just updating you about my foot surgery, now 12 weeks past. The foot has healed well, although still bothered with swelling. I am keeping it elevated and massaging it to help disperse fluid. Scar sensitivity is improving, and big toe has good mobility. According to my GP, I am experiencing biomechanical pain? I have pain and aching in right hip and lower back, also the right side of abdomen. He explained this was as a result of the body regaining correct traction after surgery and has referred me for physio.

My last review appointment is in a week's time so I may be told when consultant can proceed with the other foot.

CFP: Thanks Deborah for your important update which is appreciated. I agree with your doctor that we can alter our walking pattern and transfer stress elsewhere. Physio is an important ingredient in recovery. If you are ready for the next stage then you are indeed progressing and will have the benefit of your experience. A comparison would be most interesting. Do you think now you were happy having one done at a time or would you have preferred both operated at once?

Debbie: As much as I would have liked to have both done at once to get over with I don't know if recovery would have been more stressful. I would hope that with the second operation I would be more mindful of not over compensating with the other side, but I know this is natural and hard to avoid. I'm hoping physio will help, as pain progresses during the day due to the nature of my job.

Carly: I was diagnosed with arthritis is my left big toe and have since had a cheilectomy[58], and then follow up survey where they inject it and wiggle your toe under anaesthetic - this was probably about 2016. I still struggle to walk long distances and can't do skiing or climbing as I can't put pressure through my big toe. The doctor suggests fusing the toe as my X-ray from this week shows the cartilage is gone and the gap between the bones is significantly diminished.

---

[58] Cheilectomy is shaving the immediate bone or bunion.

Right foot: I heard a pop in March, at which point I then couldn't wriggle my toes and my foot swelled up. I have struggled to walk on the foot since as it continues to swell up and the toes don't wriggle intermittently when I walk too much. X-rays have ruled out stress fractures. They thought it was a Morton's neuroma[59] but that's been ruled out as the pain and swelling is on the top of my foot. My toes seem to separate between the second and middle toes like a V. This didn't happen before the pop. Side note - I was born flat-footed. I've requested access to my medical notes

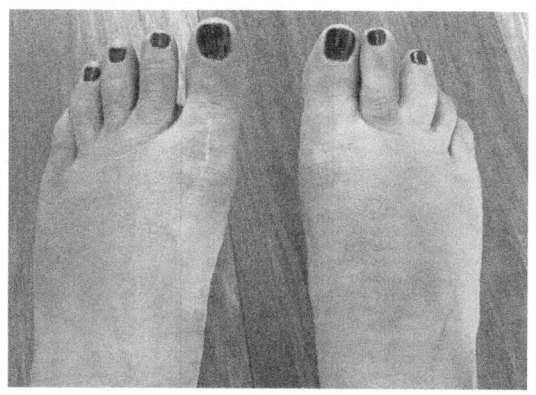

Fig.4.15 Carly's foot after surgery. Note that an incision line (scar) has been placed on top of the foot. The right foot shows a scar on the inside.

CFP: Carly, Can I ask your age? I assume you will be on your feet a lot.

Carly: I'm 35 and work in an office so not on my feet so much. I've had an ultrasound on the right foot which the operator suggested was showing a neuroma but the consultant seemed to disagree when he looked this week.

---

[59] Morton's neuroma – pinched nerve between third and fourth toes.

I'll wait and see what the MRI shows! I feel better that you would also suggest the fusion as it was something I wasn't sure would be a good idea - it doesn't sound pleasant!

CFP: Left foot / Cheilectomy conversions work best with a fusion because you may have limited bone available to work on to offer something else. It seems a reasonable suggestion to me. Right foot / there is a small gap that suggests something between the metatarsals, or you have weakened the joint, so the toe has drifted. Ultrasound is the best assessment method for neuroma or bursa, but sometimes they coexist. Pop sounds could be a joint or a neuroma moving. MRI is only partially reliable and can be open to misdiagnosis.

We have operated on a negative MRI only to find at the operation that one existed. Flat feet can play a part but are not the key concern.

Stay with your orthopaedic team if you are happy or get a second opinion. Neuroma surgery has an 83% success rate but there are other treatments which do not involve surgery but will depend on the size of the neuroma/bursa. I think you could see your surgeon. I hope this helps a little but there is no real self-treatment at this stage.

Fusions work well and if you follow the instructions then you should be okay. However ask if it is likely if you need a bone graft because a cheilectomy can be aggressive, often removing more bone than needed, although from your picture it looks minimalistic. To be honest a cheilectomy in a young person of your age or younger would not be my ideal choice as it does not last.

Ami: At fifty-one years of age and I can barely walk ten minutes. I've had surgery on both feet two years ago. *Vallux hallgus* (sic), One being two years ago and the second eighteen months now. Can you help me I was an athlete prior to surgery, and now fat, can barely do sports, and have put on weight!! [60]

CFP: Usually, if surgery has not been successful, you need to discuss this with the consultant who operated. Granted Covid may have upset matters. Have you pursued this avenue or discussed the outcome with your doctor? Not all surgery goes to plan, sadly, and dealing with problems must be carefully considered but often successful.

Sable: I'm now six weeks post-operation from my bunion surgery, and I've noticed that my big toe is significantly shorter than before surgery; it's quite noticeable in comparison to the second toe and the other foot; there is also a noticeable gap between the first and second toe. Is this normal? Will my toe go back to its normal length and will the gap between the two toes close up over time? I've been doing the exercises and joint mobility is improving daily .

---

[60] NB. Such complex case histories are not for general online solutions.

Here's a pic so you can see what I mean (so sorry my toes look wild, I haven't had a pedicure since last year.

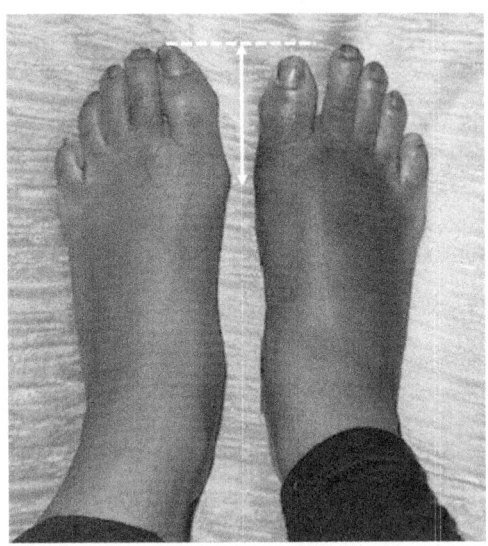

Fig.4.16. Sable's foot shows shortening on the right side following surgery.

CFP: Six weeks —Your right foot does have shortening, which is common for some procedures. The amount of bone removed relates to the extent a toe shortens. Most foot surgeons try to avoid excessive shortening, but this has to be balanced to create an effective correction. The gap closes between toes because swelling causes distortion and needs to subside. The right foot is swollen and may remain so for several months. Maintaining activity and increasing weight bearing to tolerance is helpful by shifting fluid by calf muscle movement. You seem to be doing everything that is required. The big toe's length will not change.

Sable: Thanks so much for the reply. This is so disappointing, I almost wish I never got it done because the length difference is so obvious

CFP: Perhaps Sable, it may not turn out so bad once you find you can get back to normal. I understand appearance is a big issue for people.

Amber *& Her Ganglion.*

Amber's query was missing, but the question was posed about her concerns about the bunion swelling and type of diagnostic investigations.

CFP: An MRI is appropriate as X-rays are sometimes not sensitive enough to cover all options. They are the best place to start. The MRI will take in the tendon and surrounding tissue. Protocols vary between countries, but my experience of the USA is that they are hypersensitive in undertaking tests to rule out any concerns. Soft tissue tumours are much more common than bone ones, and swelling is often just a harmless ganglion. Diclofenac sodium may help with pain, but it does not have good penetrating power. Diagnosis is essential, and surgery is not conducted until a clear picture is confirmed. An ultrasound would have also been helpful, but you should await your MRI and try not to worry, as foot cancer is rare. Undoubtedly you will get the right treatment.

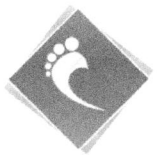

Gail's case is one of woe and frustration, under-correction, and complex problems that added to her foot condition. US spelling has not been altered.

Gail: I had bunion surgery on both feet on January 31, 2023. Both have not turned out well. I did not have much post-op care with the surgeon and was not able to get advice from him when needed. He would not even return a call from my family doctor.

My family doctor suggested I send some pictures and X-rays to ask if CFP had an opinion as to why the surgery failed, so I am attaching pictures. The doctor also requested revision surgery from a different orthopedic surgeon. The surgeon replied that he had looked at my file and saw that I had previous metatarsal osteotomy but still had significant hallux valgus, metatarsus primus varus[61] and hallux rigidus. He said he thinks the only reasonable solution to this problem would be a first MTP realignment arthrodesis, i.e. fusion and if I'm interested in this option he would see me, and he does not think a revision bunionectomy is something that he would offer. Can you tell from the picture of my X-rays why my surgery did not work, and do you think I could have revision surgery to fix it or is fusions my only option.

---

[61] Metatarsus primus varus is related to the high angle between the first and second metatarsals as shown in Part I.

I have a referral to an orthopedic surgeon that was put in by my physiatrist[62], but he had said it would take two years to get an appointment that's why I went ahead with the bunionectomy surgery in January that a different surgeon offered. Two years seemed like a long time to wait, but now it looks like I will still be dealing with my foot problems by then anyway, and I'm in way more pain now than before surgery. My family doctor says he doesn't know the answers to my questions, and I don't want to make another mistake or have fusion if my feet can be fixed. I've found with this type of surgery there are so many others like me left with so many questions and without the answers that you willingly provide. Ten to fifteen minutes in a doctor's office does not leave much time for questions and no information sheets were provided to me before or after surgery.

CFP: We have reviewed your enclosures. Thank you for the details. Sorry you've had a disappointing result. There is no doubt that your bunion surgery has not been successful, and in this regard, it appears that the surgery has not addressed the primary problem of a high intermetatarsal angle known as metatarsus primus varus. No further tests are necessary as it is quite clear from the X-rays that the operation has not achieved the purpose that it was designed for.

Seventy per cent of surgery is successful, but in 20% of cases, the surgery may under-correct where hallux valgus is large. However, overall 5 to 10% of surgery can be unsuccessful. The reason for this is that the deformity is

---

[62] A physiatrist is a medical doctor (USA) who specialises in physical medicine and rehabilitation. They treat conditions of the bones, muscles, joints, brain, and nervous system.

challenging for the surgeon, or the surgeon may not have sufficient experience in dealing with such a deformity or able to offer a range of different procedures.

The MAAS procedure was the correct title; MOHS was misleading, unfortunately.

You will have to have revision surgery almost certainly because you will be disappointed with the positioning, and the joint may continue to be painful. You have consulted a second surgeon, and the recommendation is for an arthrodesis which on balance, is the safer option. The toe will remain stiff and affect certain shoes in terms of the heel height you can comfortably wear. This means there will be some permanency in restricting shoe selection. Revision surgery carries a risk of further shortening the first metatarsal, which can lead to pain under the ball of the foot. It should be avoided because there is a definite risk, which could be as high as 25%.

It is always desirable to provide as detailed information prior to surgery as possible. Do contact the surgeon for further advice. Breakdown in communications is a common disappointment. The previous surgeon you saw for a second opinion would almost certainly be right to recommend a fusion. Take a little time considering this before stepping into further surgery to allow everything to resolve as best as possible, just in case you feel that you can live with what you have.

(Gail's long response showed the emotional side of her treatment and care in the USA.)

CFP: We must point out that there are very few surgeons, including ourselves, who have not had problems following surgery, so perfection is never guaranteed in anyone's hands Long-term may become unsatisfactory if left untreated. It would be best to give the foot a little time to settle before embarking on further surgery. Find someone you can trust.

If you plan to have further surgery, the surgeon or anaesthetist should provide you with what we call a regional block, which will freeze the whole limb for 24 hours if possible. Ordinary painkillers are also added, but after the limb is essentially frozen, you will not feel the need for these.

When the first metatarsal surgery fails, there are only two approaches left. You can either live with the condition or have further surgery. Revision surgery requires the metatarsal to be lengthened, and this does need to be done by someone with expertise and prior experience.

The second surgeon you saw was not keen on revision surgery because of the complexity, and he is at least recognising his limitations. For this reason, he has suggested fusing the toe, which is a safer bet because, generally, these are successful despite losing range of movement. The correction from this procedure is usually encouraging. The recovery from the arthrodesis procedure is around six weeks, although all surgery takes longer for swelling to reduce with full recovery at 6-9 months. The revision surgery could take a baseline of 4 months and has an element of risk that requires a year to recover from. That risk does include failure for the bone to heal or complete alignment to be achieved. Revision surgery must aim at lengthening the bone and correcting the metatarsus primus angle, which has, in fact, not been corrected.

You can appreciate that these two elements are critical to a satisfactory outcome. You make special mention of the need to cut more bone. Revision surgery requires bone placed into the existing metatarsal to compensate for the loss of length.

This bone has to be harvested either from somewhere else or your own body, which adds to the complexity of the operation. You can now see why this becomes a highly specialised operation.

Spacers that hold the toe apart can prove comfortable. Without surgery, there is no solution for an under-corrected toe deformity, so you cannot rely on spacers to resolve the toe position. Likewise, physiotherapy can only help improve the range of movement up to a certain level but will not correct the toe. Books written with false promises that bunions can be corrected without surgery are misleading. Footwear will become challenging, and getting the right length and width. You have a better range of footwear in the United States of America than we do in the UK, which might give you a better option. You could elect to have shoes made to measure, but this adds to the overall cost of your medical care.

(Gail's reply was full of gratitude, but she had medical problems that necessitated considerable support and understanding.)

Lois: Dear CFP, I would appreciate any advice you could offer. Below is a picture of my foot six weeks after scarf[63] akin surgery. It was intensely painful with marked redness. Shooting pains continued for many months. I had three pins and a cast. Fig.4.18.

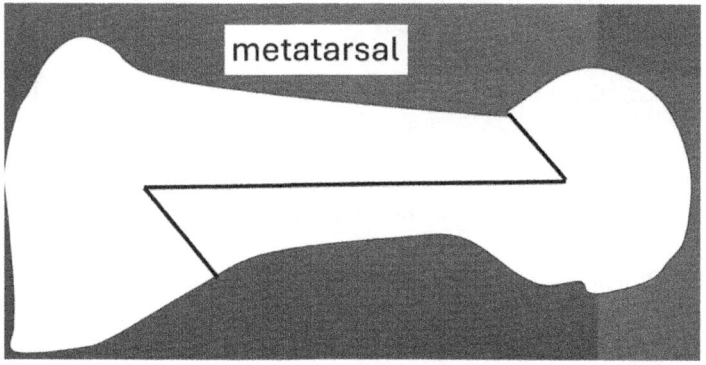

metatarsal

Fig. 4.17. Scarf osteotomy is based on a stable carpentry cut that offers earlier mobility. (See Fig 4.8 for Akin).

Now, ten months after surgery, I have what feels like a tight elastic band around my toes and an uncomfortable feeling that I am standing on a pebble under the base of my big toe. My big toe is still raised off the ground, although my foot is not swollen.

I had a X-ray a couple months ago which shows the toe is now angulating back to pre op position which I know can

---

[63] Scarf osteotomy can be viewed on YouTube. https://www.youtube.com/watch?v=knVqJa9vlu8

happen and as I have hypermobile joints my podiatrist says surgery failure is even more likely. I am due to have a steroid injection in a couple of weeks, but I am not sure whether it will help. I don't want to risk ending up in any worse position.

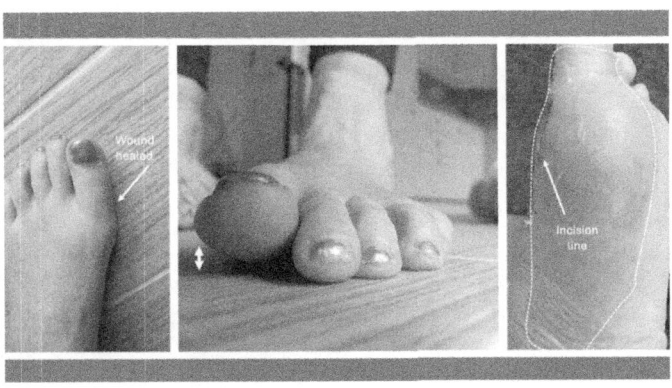

Fig.4.18. Lois provided pictures of her foot to enable CFP to gain an idea of her problem.

CFP: The foot is not swollen and has no high colour in the post-operative image. The alignment is certainly not optimal for a scarf-akin, but often, a small amount of regression does not trouble patients, that is, if there is an improvement overall. Patients all react differently after surgery. Your surgeon will have ruled out infection, so the only other reason for continuing pain could be a reaction to the metalwork. This is rare but not unheard of. Broken hardware (I am assuming screws rather than pins) should have shown up by X-ray, although even broken hardware can be ignored if it has not moved. How do we know if it is a hardware reaction - well, the best method is to remove it all.

The second cause of continuous pain is a nerve condition

called complex regional pain syndrome (CRPS). This causes redness and colour changes with temperature fluctuations in the foot, swelling and sensitivity to light touch. You have not revealed any of this, but a competent surgeon should be able to advise you if CRPS is present.

If all avenues have been followed, there is sometimes no resolution other than permanently stiffening the toe so it does not move at the joint. I would only recommend this option, called an arthrodesis if movement at the joint is painful. The fact that the toe sits higher and affects purchase is down to the surgical alignment that can arise. It does affect shoe fit in some designs. While most bunion surgeries settle and are successful, in 25-30% of cases, results are less ideal, with less than 5% going on to cause distressing concerns.

Many people seek a second opinion at this stage, but if you have confidence in your surgeon, stay in touch with him/her and have a 12-month review. If you can find a way to accommodate the problem and avoid actively causing pain, that is a solution, but one where you, the patient, must accept surgery has left limitations. I know this is far from ideal, and second surgeries have been known to make matters worse.

Loose Ends & Tips

The diaries and correspondence illustrate a broad selection of problems. When combined, there are areas of overlap, but in the final analysis, we need to draw some of these problems together.

Days 1–40 typify most journeys, with 6–8 weeks for recovery, but it can take longer depending on the type of surgery. The question might well be posed: what is recovery? Recovery is not about wound healing but the fact you can re-engage with your pre-surgical life.

- The ability to ability to wear shoes.
- Returning to your occupation full-time or part-time.
- Sporting activities and hobbies can be resumed.
- Engage in all social activities.

Recovery is perceived by the patient, not by the clinician. This was more unusual when one female patient returned to her occupation as a fitness instructor at two weeks. An audit of cases from the Royal College of Podiatry suggests footwear return takes 6-8 weeks, but some outliers take longer.

Slippers, sandals and Wellington boots are not usual footwear but may be better tolerated because they create less pressure and allow swelling.

- Dressing check: Try to stay with the clinic/hospital that treats you for consistency.
- Sleeping: If possible, use separate beds and, in the early days, create a foot cradle from a cardboard box, turned upside down with a cut out for the foot and leg.
- Getting help: Make sure you have the correct numbers for out-of-hours assistance. Use the emergency number given rather than visit an A&E department. Do so early rather than late in the day.
- Returning to work: Be honest with your employer, but only return after the recommended period.
- Aids and safety: The shoes provided will accommodate dressings. Crutches are essential for the first week. Aircast boots allow better stability and improve movement safety. Return to all activities slowly and follow guided information.
- Dealing with pain: Use medications early, but let staff know if you have allergies, problems with constipation, nausea, or dizziness.
- Infection: It usually does not show up for 48+ hours, more often on Day 4 or later. Note if pain increases despite taking analgesics. Seek advice from the surgical unit.
- Showers and dressings: Do not shower for 48 hours; use recommended shower covers only. Safety is essential in a shower, and accidents like broken bones can arise.
- Colour changes are common and can last for many months but subside.
- Swelling: Except where a blood clot happens, swelling diminishes by four months but can continue for twelve months.

- Exercises and weight gain: Weight gain is an unwanted byproduct of non-movement.
- Non-weight-bearing exercises can be used, especially lying on your back.
- Food selection and quantity are important during the early days, especially if eating is linked with boredom.

Elevation of Leg & Foot

CASE STUDY: Positive elevation

When called to a patient's house for pain management, the effects of elevating her leg reduced her pain immediately. Icing can help reduce pain by up to 40%. Foot position is vital. Place cushions, blankets or foam under the thigh. Bend the knee – avoid crushing the calf muscle, but support the foot in this position at the ankle tendon (Achilles). Elevation is used largely for periods when pain or swelling is greatest. It is not necessary all of the time.

CASE STUDY: Downside of elevation

Puzzled by a patient who phoned in to tell me she had a numb heel after surgery, her outstretched leg had pulled the long sciatic nerve. At its thickest the nerve is the same diameter as the small finger. Bend the leg at the knee with the leg still raised to overcome this problem.

Unreasonable Employers

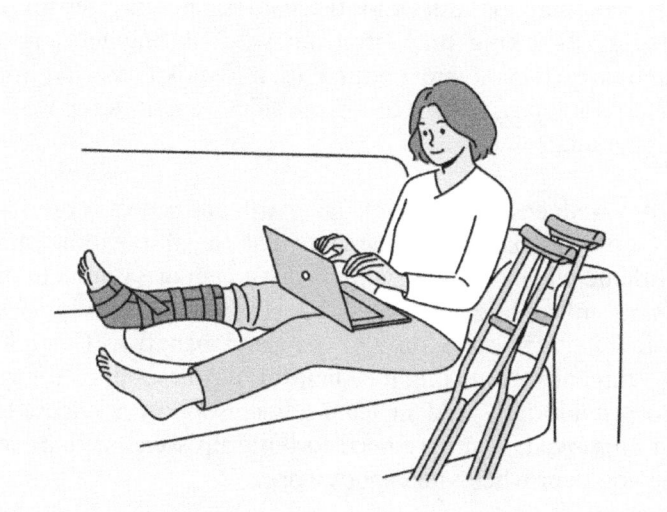

Work & Your Occupation

'It's only a bunion. Why do you need to be off so long?'
'We need you here. Get back as soon as you can. I'm sure you won't need that long!'

These are real words from uncaring organisations, which amount to bullying. Although it is not covered in her diary journey, one patient did have problems at work. Here are a few tips.

Your surgeon can suggest in a letter how long you should be off your feet and when you should return to duties. Many patients use their holiday to ease the burden, and where possible, consultants will try and accommodate this. Teachers perhaps fall into the largest holiday-sensitive category as taking time off from work during term is a nightmare. If you are entitled to a requisite period for sickness and pay, work it in so both sides benefit. Keep work on your side.

Income reduces with the time taken off, and repeat surgeries can affect sickness entitlement. The legal position and entitlements change constantly, so we cannot say much on this as information needs to be current. All workplaces should have policies on sick pay and benefits. The UK government website might be helpful[64]. Your employer may also provide independent legal advice/support services. If self-employed, you may need to build up some savings to tide you over when you cannot work.

Don't be unrealistic with time off work. Bunion surgery takes 6–8 weeks to recover from as a generalisation. We have seen some patients return to work within two weeks and others unable to return to work full-time for sixteen weeks. If you give work an unrealistic return date, you set yourself up for a problem. A second unscheduled period of work absence adds to potential penalisation. Some employers have stringent rules about how many days are allowed before staff are disciplined. Take the right amount of time off, and do not short-circuit it.

---

[64] https://www.gov.uk/taking-sick-leave Accessed September 2024.

CASE STUDY

A teacher had bunion surgery, returned to work and at six weeks, sat down in floods of tears when attending a follow-up appointment. It transpired she had been bullied to go back earlier than she should have. She was expected to stand and walk distances between classrooms, encounter flights of stairs and risk young children treading on her foot. There is only one response: you now need more time off work, extending the original time. Working out time needed off from work is not easy, complex bunion surgeries may need 10–12 weeks.

FIT FOR WORK – A GUIDE

You can go back to work provided that you:

Can you walk half a mile comfortably.

Have reasonable stability in the great toe.

Do not need anything more for pain relief than a random paracetamol or ibuprofen (nothing stronger).

Sleep reasonably well at night.

Can drive for an hour safely in control, without distraction from pain.

You can wear shoes appropriate for wet and cold weather.

Can stand for 30–45 minutes without suffering more than minor swelling.

Have a wound that has healed and is strong enough for daily activity without risk of breakdown.

Have no scabs or dried crusty areas by Week 6.

Do not have any open wounds.

If you have a sedentary job behind a desk or counter, you should be able to sit, which is fine. If you have a more active job, you must be cautious about early return. If you work in an industry with equipment, are exposed to higher-risk elements, drive long distances, or need to use heavy-duty boots, you will need longer to ensure you are fit for duty. Fitness to work is important. While your employer should ensure you can work safely, they must be clear about what you can and cannot do. Return to work is better graduated and shows that a company or organisation is truly sensitive towards its employees.

Early return is an advantage from the psychological point of view, i.e. feeling useful again and being busy. Occupational health departments support staff return to work so repatriation can be positive and supportive throughout—some of the best employers in helping employees include the police force and NHS in the UK. It is reasonable that your workplace understands the nature of the surgery and the immobilisation needed. A husband who posted a photograph of his wife on social media caused a problem:

> [I was] using a motability scooter to get around the store, with the subsequent picture being posted to social media by my husband. This picture then caused certain colleagues to question my need to still be off work as I was now going out!

If you are bullied into returning earlier than recommended, be clear that this is against medical care recommendations. Your GP and the consultant will support you, and you are entitled to any notes that reflect this view. Bullying is counterproductive, and any employee disadvantaged after surgery should raise this at a higher managerial level through occupational health and inform their medical/allied health team of the problem.

Glossary of Key Areas Following Surgery

Aids to Walking and Safety

Crutches should be fitted to ensure the right arm–leg length balance. A badly adjusted crutch is likely to cause back pain and falls. It is important to lay down ground rules that exclude using crutches as weapons, tools, props or taking excess weight. A damaged crutch can also cause the patient to collapse if the metal fatigues. The rubber stop on the bottom (ferrule) should not be worn down – do not use old crutches borrowed from people. Two crutches are often preferred to widen your base and remove pressure from the injured side, but take advice from the discharging team. Pain can arise in many joints where it should not if poorly used without guidance. Many prefer sticks, and there is nothing wrong with this, but perhaps not in the early stages of recovery from bunion surgery.

Getting out is good, but do it safely.

'Two feet' surgery patients do best with wheelchairs in the first week to allow safe mobility and respite, as crutches can be exhausting after both feet have been operated on— reserve places ahead of time in theatres, cinemas, or similar events with large numbers of people. Check out seat plans early to avoid disappointment. The ultimate support for foot surgery comes in the form of a leg-supported on a scooter.

Shopping and leaving home safely can contribute to a healthy recovery. These systems are available for hire during the recovery period.

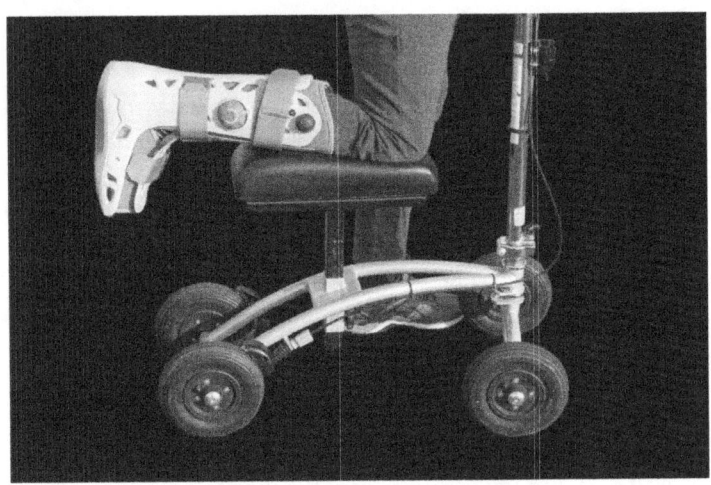

Fig.4.20. Knee scooter allows greater mobility with safety. Shown with an air boot.

Cast and foot/ankle immobilisation

Special post-op shoes are designed to take a thick dressing, which would not otherwise fit into a regular shoe. A wedge shoe is heavier and allows offloading of the front of the foot. Like most forms of aid, this lifts one side of the body and can cause back and hip problems if overused. This is highlighted in the diary journeys. Velcro straps allow adjustability, but once the dressing comes off, the shoe is looser and ordinary sandals are better as the dressings become lighter.

An air cast boot is a substitute and can be used from days 4–10 onwards. Our patient, Rose, highlights the AircastTM boot's effect on posture and joints, such as the hip and back.

The cast boot can be used during the day, removed at rest, and for icing the foot, showering, and sleeping. A strap can be adjusted at different levels around the foot, ankle and leg for security. An inflatable bladder within the system allows air to be pumped into the cast so it fits snugly. Ensuring the right size is vital to prevent rubbing. A gel bunion shield can protect the wound inside the boot joint, making the foot more comfortable and helpfully compressing the scar. Used too early, however, this can make the wound sweat, particularly in summer months. The shield is available online and from some high street outlets.

Bedclothes

Nighttime is a big concern for many – bedclothes can place pressure on the operated foot. There is no need to buy a bed cage when a cardboard box would do. Cut out one side of a stiff box about 50–60cm high (Fig.4.20). This allows the foot to slide in so the bed sheets can sit on top. Jo commented (P.136) about sleeping in bed as she was worried about her partner knocking her foot. We tend to sleep poorly as we age and become fidgety after surgery, and worry about the foot being knocked. Separate beds are a good idea for healing.

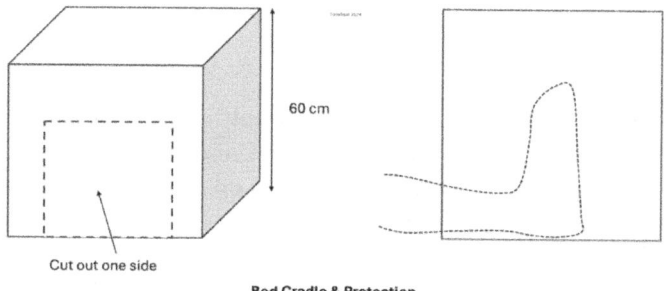

60 cm

Cut out one side

Bed Cradle & Protection

Fig. 4.20.

Whiling Away the Hours (at home)

Support networks can range from social media to friends, neighbours and family. Be careful, though: if you are off work on sick leave and seen out, it may be interpreted as your being fit to work. Rose, Florinda and Jackie developed their own strategy to occupy their idle hours. There are only so many daytime TV or radio programmes you can watch or listen to, books (or Kindles) you can read, Sudokus, and crosswords you can puzzle over – not least as the repetitive position makes us uncomfortable. Having a comfy place in the house is important and Rose was magnetised to her snug with good garden views. She offered wonderful descriptions that I have edited out as brevity required many such descriptions to be trimmed. Rose was well organised, and in her case children did not factor in. Rose and Jackie also had previous experience, whereas for Florinda, this was her first experience; even she felt out of her depth.

Although animals can provide distraction and emotional support, they can also trample over a painful foot. Even after surgery, it is easy to hammer the injured foot with further injury, something that Jackie and Florinda managed. A jet-wash machine was going a bit too far, let alone a full two-litre bottle of fizz!

Getting Help

Out-of-office-hours-help is important and out-of-hours contact numbers will be provided on discharge sheets. Avoid A&E as they will not be interested unless you have a life-threatening condition. GPs are still the first line if your surgical service cannot see you quickly, but they will only stabilise and assess the urgency.

Jackie went to her GP service then onto a community-based hospital, so used a range of help networks. In the independent sector a resident medical officer (RMO) is employed as a liaison between patients and consultant, but the ward and physiotherapy department may all work to provide support as consultants, or attendings as in the USA, Surgeons are not resident or keep daily hours.

Outside office hours, the ward takes the call. During office hours outpatient nursing responds and then refers on to the RMO if the concern needs escalating. The nurse and RMO can contact the consultant for advice or discuss treatment or even call the consultant in, depending upon the problem

Patient-induced Problems

While most bunion surgeries go well, a few have problems. Many sort themselves out, but a few become nightmares. Meryl and Jess are examples of two worst-case scenarios.

CASE STUDY: Sun precautions

Meryl's foot split wide open after sunbathing. The wound was wider after delayed healing took place. Returning to theatre after primary surgery is challenging for all parties.

CASE STUDY: Smoking

Jess smoked, doubling her usual smoking from 15 to 30 cigarettes a day after feeling imprisoned in the house. Jess's foot deteriorated and necessitated two trips back to theatre as her healing was affected by the nicotine and other products in cigarettes. After five months she had no movement because of scarring.

Pain Management

Surgery usually creates an element of pain. Our case study diaries illustrate a variety of periods when discomfort arose. Damage to nerve endings and inflammation will cause signs and symptoms. This is normal. We aim to minimise that pain experience, but pain is not a disadvantage—it forces us to slow down so we can repair tissue safely.

Modern surgery involves local anaesthetics called regional anaesthetic blocks. These are effectively placed around the ankle or even as high as the knee. Extending pain control to 24-hours is achievable today because of new anaesthetic agents and accuracy and placement of the drug.

Rose found she was on a high until the block wore off. Florinda did less well and was in pain the next morning as she had not slept. If Florinda had been at home it could have been a great deal more worrying without experienced nursing available. Both Rose and Jackie had pain once a wound problem emerged. The pain was an indicator that something needed further attention. These were low-impact concerns but required time and patience to settle. The timescales may appear long in both reported cases, but the wound healing and recovery was not unusual.

Opiates/opioids

The group of medications called opiates (derived from the opium poppy, like heroin) are perhaps the most powerful method of relieving pain that we know. Most people appreciate the fact that opiates cause addiction, but when used short term and for their intended purpose, addiction is rare if not unlikely. The lowest UK strength of codeine is 8mg and can be bought over the counter with supervision from an attendant pharmacist.

These drugs can be mixed with paracetamol (*Tylenol* (acetaminophen) in the US). On its own the drug works for mild-to-moderate pain only and is not ideal for bunion surgery.

The group called the non-steroidal anti-inflammatories, or NSAIDs, include ibuprofen and are not opioids. These work differently and have a better effect on reducing inflammation after surgery. Paracetamol and ibuprofen work well for more than 70% of patients but some will need codeine. As the dose of the opioid rises, so do the potential side effects. If you are taking opiates you can fall over easily, especially when dizzy. Jackie wrestled with this problem.

Tramadol is preferred for stronger pain relief. Morphine and strong codeine given as two tablets at 30mg strength (60mg) can cause disorientation and lower blood pressure. In the case of Florinda this upset her bowel movements. Opioids slow down the muscles in the bowel and affect the water content, so the stool becomes harder and has a longer passage through the gut. The strain put through the end muscles (anal wall) is affected and it can be sore on evacuating a solid stool. The bowel develops varicose veins, which are weakened through repeated straining and lead to haemorrhoids (piles). Piles can bleed and are then visible. Itchiness and general discomfort may require treatment. Dark or light blood stains appear alarming on toilet paper or the stool.

Constipation

To avoid constipation, you have to take the long view. Pain over constipation or constipation over pain? If your pain is controlled, avoid all pain medication except for those twilight zones; the first 36–48 hours as described by the diaries.

Use any low-dose drug that does not cause the problem. Ibuprofen can still cause constipation but it can also cause diarrhoea as well. Keeping hydrated is important but not to the extent you are needing to relieve yourself every hour. If your blood pressure is low, you may be on a drip; this tends to occur with general anaesthetic rather than local anaesthetic.

Laxatives are used to offset constipation. The use of fibre gel and sugary medications like lactulose may help, or *Senokot* (senna) and bisacodyl (e.g. *Dulcolax*) can be bought from the pharmacist (if not prescribed for you). Prunes and high-fibre foods are good and modern juicing techniques allow easier ingestion by mixing prunes with pears. Some laxatives can upset diabetes so ask advice from your local pharmacist. Avoid eating red meat before surgery and stay with a high-fibre diet. Bear in mind everyone is different. Sometimes, there is no way around constipation, but if you do have significant bowel problems, it is best to have a discussion with your physician (GP) or a specialist in this area.

Cryotherapy and icing the foot

Here are a few hints about ice (cryotherapy). Most centres will provide ice packs, while many prefer the mouldability and utility of frozen peas. Special jackets exist, such as those produced by Aircast™, which are higher tech. Bunion surgery patients provided with cryotherapy jackets found this contributed to effective pain management. Reducing swelling (oedema) helps reduce nerve activity. Elevating the foot and leg helps relieve throbbing and tightness.

Ice, of course, has its risks

A foot that is too cool for too long may develop frostbite. This arises with older patients and those with poor peripheral circulation and thin, fragile skin.

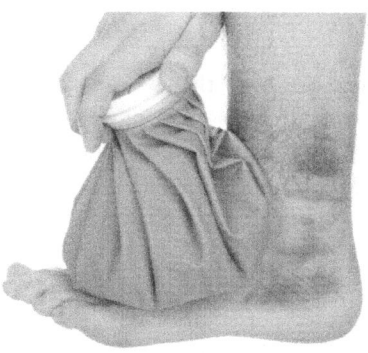

Fig.4.21. A useful method of applying crushed ice safely. Avoid placing directly over the surgical site.

A Quick Guide To Icing

Do not ice directly over the wound.
Ice should be kept away from the surgical site.
Cooling at the back of the foot rather than over the wound directly.
Ice jackets may be safer than direct ice from the freezer.
Jackets applied over thicker dressings can be left longer than thin coverings.
The length of use is probably around 10–20 minutes at a time, with a 40–60-minute gap between sessions.
More pain, more ice perhaps – with care for the skin (as above).

Healing And Wounds

Infection and surgical site

Redness increases, and the wound swells and becomes painful. The wound may open and produce a thin or thick discharge. If the odour becomes unpleasant, this indicates further deterioration and a need for assistance. The dressing may have a heavier discharge that seeps through. Sticky discharge adds to the problem and can indicate some cell death, which needs cleaning. Oral antibiotics are needed early if red streaks arise toward the ankle and leg. Pain behind the knee or groin is a sign of a spreading infection. Consider this an emergency to avoid becoming ill. Cellulitis is when the foot balloons split and discharge. Toxins need to be treated with intravenous antibiotics and probably hospitalisation if the body temperature rises.

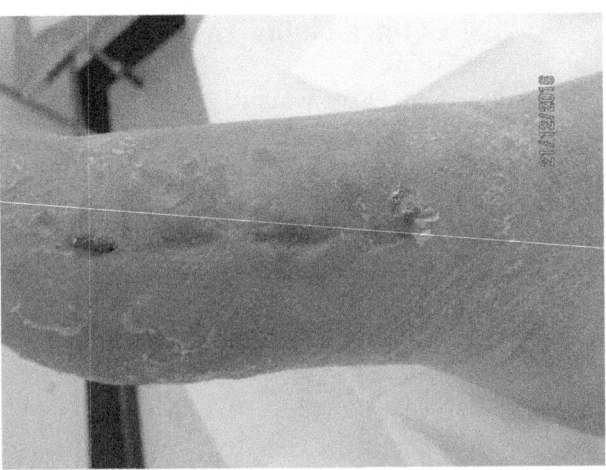

Fig.4.22. Wounds that cause delayed recovery, sometimes require surgical intervention.

Surgical cleaning (debridement)

The length of time a moist (macerated) wound takes to heal can vary as the lower layers have to produce new healing elements. Pain eases once a small covering of cells has occurred, but the foot may itch and slowly mend. Sometimes surgery is necessary to clean the damaged tissue that fails to heal, as seen in Meryl and Jess's case studies. Surgery consists of washing and scraping (debridement) the damaged element to restore a better blood supply. Wounds are usually left open without sutures. There is a longer delay in healing with open wounds.

Blisters

Bleeding, blisters and maceration are all mentioned in the diaries and are worth discussing further.

Jackie and Rose had different problems. So you may ask how long it takes to heal a wound after bunion surgery. Skin is made of two distinct layers. The top (epidermis) is waterproof, the bottom layer (dermis) carries the chief ingredients like tiny blood vessels and nerves. The two layers sit on a further layer of fat. If you have studied biology at any level you will realise it is not quite that simple, but anyone who has cut themselves with a knife knows it takes little time for the top layer to join together if the cut is simple and not jagged. The cut will heal provided it is not too hot or wet. Dressings are designed to absorb blood or the thinner seepage (exudate), which slows down as the blood hardens, forming a scab. The scab is made of hardened blood cells called platelets and prevents bleeding, but it can be easily knocked in the early stages. The scab braces the wound and helps to heal the wound unless it widens.

Stitches and Tapes

Most surgery involves internal, absorbing stitches (sutures), but the weakness is that skin can open if stressed. Too much activity or sudden bleeding will cause this premature opening. The incision on the side of the foot offers less visible exposure than if placed on the top of the toe joint, but has the disadvantage of being exposed to side pressure. Wounds that follow a normal pattern are clean and well aligned at 7–14 days[65] and on their way to healing by 3–6 weeks. Full strength allegedly firms up by six months and the scar contracts over two years.

Steristrips are used as thin tapes to stop the skin opening when a dissolving suture is used. If this becomes moist it needs removing. On Day 9, Jackie had her problem revealed. She was already struggling badly with over-strong pain medication: as she rightly said, her dizziness was due to her sensitivity to codeine.

If the top layer becomes heated and sweaty, as in Jackie's case, the strength is lost and has to be repaired. The layers peel away (sloughing), and nerve endings have heightened sensitivity and are less comfortable.

Continuity of care from skilled staff is important and varies in GP practices because of different experiences and exposure to surgical wounds. Jackie was right to return to the hospital, where surgery was carried out, but she did have appropriate care once the wound showed signs of deteriorating. By Day 20, she records that things were better and she had 'turned the corner'. This suggests her problem arose over eleven days.

---

[65] Times in days for healing are generalisations only. Some people will take longer than others.

Nausea and Headaches

Nausea can arise from low fluid intake. This happens less as we understand the body's processes, such as giving fluid during surgery. This is not necessary with local anaesthetic, as the body has less disturbance and minimal frequency of headaches, as well as reduced necessity to starve before admission. Medications given at the time of surgery will help to minimise the effect. If you know that you suffer nausea, it is a good idea to talk to both the surgeon and anaesthetist so a regional anaesthetic block can be used.

Showers, Dressings and Recovery

There are some general tips and guides associated with this subject. The first is to keep the wound dry. If wet or soggy, make sure the dressing is changed immediately and ideally return to have this changed if the problem arises within days of surgery. Do not attempt to shower for two days. Why? You have just had surgery, and in terms of complexity, hallux valgus-bunion surgery is not minor, even if it was a day case. Problems following surgery often arise when patients need to follow instructions.

Use a seat in the shower and ensure help for a bath from a relative or partner. Protect the foot with a sleeve that reaches above the knee. The Limbo cover is a reliable product. A plastic bag sealed with tape does not guarantee a dry dressing inside. Often, a patient has turned up with a soggy dressing, having tried to save money by using plastic bags that let water in. The Limbo cover is reinforced and has a neoprene gasket. Water will not enter the bag if the shower head is not directly over the elasticated opening. The main advantage of investing in a cover is its reusable nature, although it can tear. As this device is needed for 10–21 days, it is worth purchasing.

Dressings are left on to protect the wound. A separating medium is incorporated to reduce the chance of the gauze sticking to the wound. This works sometimes but not all the time. Once left to the air, any skin wound, if clean (no bugs), will dry and do well. A scab is evident and will disappear within six weeks, leaving a pink trench.

Once the wound heals, you can start massaging the foot, compressing the soft tissue and forcing the fluid back toward the ankle to be carried away by the drainage vessels (lymphatics and veins). Massage and careful exercise will improve the colour and discourage unwanted reflex pain sensations after foot surgery, aiding the scar to soften and making the area less lumpy. Tethering produced by a deep scar is minimised.

Colour changes after surgery

Most of us are unaware that even after a small skin injury, the wound alters in many ways. Skin colour changes temporarily after foot surgery. Bruising arises from escaped blood content, which can migrate to the heel or arch and may appear well away from the surgery site. There is no need for concern as this bruising will soon disappear.

General redness or even purple colour may take longer to disappear. This can vary during the day, after rest, or even after having a warm shower or bath. The healing process is complex as there is mass disturbance at all levels. The colour reflects the state of the small vessels (capillaries) and the larger conducting blood vessels – arterioles or arteries – which change diameter through reflex controls and repair as they may have been cut and cauterised.

Cold makes the skin pale or blue, and heat makes the skin darker or red after surgery as the circulatory status is temporarily altered for months, not just weeks.

Much can be done to improve the foot's colour, which occasionally appears alarming. Drop the foot down, and the colour will change dramatically. Elevate the limb, and the foot's colour will improve. Rest and elevation are important during the first week after surgery. Still, as comfort returns, exercises like muscle pumping are valuable, not just to prevent a venous blood clot (DVT).

How long should swelling last?

Swelling— (oedema [UK]/edema [US]) limits movement and is normal. But how long should swelling last? There is no magic figure in weeks or months. Think of a figure and double it, but you still might be wrong. Swelling is a process that remains permanent in some rare cases, although certainly not dramatically. Legs with inefficient veins or a poor drainage system (lymph) can cause problems. The main downside of the first toe is swelling under the first metatarsal, which causes the toe to stick up. This is not uncommon but dies down after a few months. The forefoot improves by the fourth month, but it is not unusual for patients to wait 9–12 months. Of course, there are outlier patients who seem to have little swelling. Using non-weight-bearing exercises can reduce swelling where the calf and thigh muscles are activated. Alternatively, an elasticated tubular bandage may help, provided the tension is not too great and causes pain. Squeezing well-established swelling in tissue is unhelpful and not ideal as the circulation can also be impaired. The aim is to build up from non-weight bearing to weight bearing.

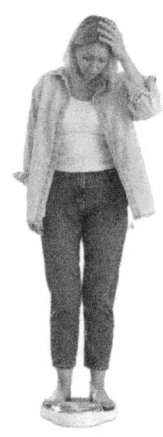

Fig.4.23. Weight gain is associated with lack of activity and eating more food than required. Maintain a good nutritional balance and avoiding high calorific intake with carbohydrates and processed sugars is important.

Weight gain and inactivity

Any period of immobility will reduce activity. Jackie understood the effects, and Florinda decided to use a programme she found online. Together with reduced activity there is boredom, and eating helps, so we graze and eat more than usual. This extra calorific load has disadvantages. For those keen on regular exercise, ceasing activity turns off the well-being hormones called endorphins. Awareness of food – the type and portion size – can assist in reducing weight gain after surgery. Avoid dependence on take-away food but DO prepare smaller portions of ready-cooked and frozen meals for the microwave. Alcohol is a weight gainer and should be minimised. Exercises include leg pedalling in the air, sit-ups and upper-body exercises. Anything you can do to keep the leg muscles working and the heart pumping faster will help reduce the risk of a blood clot, as the blood is kept moving under higher pressures.

Has This Book Achieved Its Aim?

You have read an analysis of what a bunion is and how it is distinguished from hallux valgus but often arises together, creating compound problems of skin, joint and nail pain. Hallux valgus may present in its rigid form—hallux valgo-rigidus. More people live with these conditions than require surgery, although it might be fair to suggest some would benefit but have an abiding fear of operations.

Self-help may only work for some, and professional assistance may be preferred depending on the type of problem. Foot health practitioners and podiatrists can manage nails—complex skin problems by podiatrists and surgery by podiatric or orthopaedic surgeons. Bespoke footwear (made to measure) has fallen from popularity due to rising costs, but there are now options for wide-fitting feet and the ability to purchase two different sizes. The choice of surgery requires careful selection between an osteotomy and an arthrodesis. Both are successful, but the longevity of correction remains variable.

Young people should defer surgery as long as possible. The use of replacement joints likewise has a finite period of life, and we have seen replacements last from 2-20 years, depending upon activity. Generally, these are used for damaged joints that might offer some but limited movement afterwards. We have always found considerable debate surrounding a need to have movement or not. Most movement in unfused joints will return by twelve months, but this can continue, as we have seen in one case study where, after three years, 60° was measured.

Consent is a tricky area—what was said, understood, and provided in writing. Where surgeries have failed to meet expectations, naturally, as we have seen in the patient messages, the disappointment is keenly felt. The route to litigation often fails because our hopes from surgery, when not met, give us a sense that something must have gone wrong.

Upon Reflection

Dr Richard Gordon was one the earliest British medical authors in the 20th century who lifted the lid of medicine for an audience mystified by its peculiarities of activities —far from a comedy, patients today have become empowered to make decisions with their doctors and health professionals.

'How different in my early days, when you didn't have to tell people what was wrong with them, you just told them what was good for them. And sent 'em away with a flea in their ear if they dared to ask any questions.'
Richard Gordon —Doctor on the Boil, 1970

We believe that few doctors, clinicians or surgeons seek to mislead patients, but in the past, medical approaches attempted to soften many aspects of treatment. Such an approach removed some elements of choice and hid many of the complications that could arise. A condition might have a 2% risk, but if that risk carried a 90% chance of disablement after treatment, then that 2% risk would be seen differently by some.

A typical response patients mentioned after being told about risks could come down to— 'I can't be any worse than I am now.' Sadly, sometimes, this is a false expectation. Hopefully, this book will go some way in ensuring that choice is not only provided but explained.

We have tried to use our experience to reflect on many cases, most of which have passed without concern and have been resolved with additional care. The detailed effects of surgery, unwanted and usual, have been provided to extend your choice. If you had read this book before entering any treatment plan, you now have more information than the websites, the Internet, and information leaflets offer.

Whatever your destination, we hope you are better off with this book than without it. Please tell others about this guidebook and leave comments on Amazon books. You can write to David at busypencilcasecfp@gmail.com.

Acknowledgements

An army, mainly patients, was required to produce this book after five years of patient correspondence. Those who wrote to 'Consultingfootpain' bared their souls and concerns to benefit those who could not ask questions—we are grateful.

A special mention was made to Sue, Selina Z, Julie, Jane, Rachel, and Rod for their original diaries, which offer such detail.

To our friends and colleagues who have reviewed this book and believed in the objectivity of producing such a guide.

Foreword writer Tony Maher, Reviewers—David Holland, Bill Liggins, Martin McGeough, Nicola Harvey, Sid Gibson and Sahiba Atwal.

To those on David's Facebook page (@davidtollafield, who assisted with the cover design our thanks and to the focus group, Paul, Jan, and Jill, who waded through numerous samples.

Petya Tsankova, as always brilliant, coped with the various cover rejections and modifications.

Original copy editors Selina Class and Stephen Finney – know that much found in the first edition has been used where it gained the greatest value.

To The Institute of Podiatrists, College of Foot Health and Royal College of Podiatry for supporting this book.

Finally, I thank my co-author, Tim, who has always been an inspiration during my post-clinical writing years.

The Authors

About the Authors

David R Tollafield

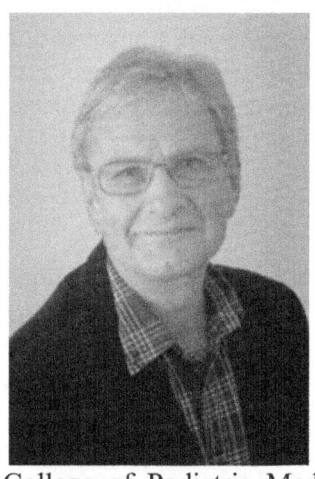

Qualified from University College Hospital (London Foot Hospital) in 1978, David worked in the community before becoming a full-time lecturer at the University of Northampton (formerly Nene College) in 1985. His early post-diploma training took him to the USA, where the Churchill Foundation Award and Silver Jubilee sponsorship allowed him to study clinical biomechanics at the California College of Podiatric Medicine for three months (1981). Later, in Seattle, at 5th Avenue Hospital (1990), he worked in the surgery department for six weeks on two rotations. He graduated in Remedial Health Science from the University of Coventry (1990), completing his surgical Fellowship in 1986. In 2016 he added his Master's degree from the University of Huddersfield. In 1995, he was awarded the consultant position in podiatric surgery for Walsall NHS Trust, which merged with the community trust. He remained in his final years within the orthopaedic directorate before leaving to work in the independent sector.

David worked in various hospitals within the West Midlands over twenty-five years and retired, becoming a full-time author with Busypencilcase Communications in 2018.

The Royal College of Podiatry awarded him the Meritorious Award for his contributions to the profession and, in 2016, the Fellowship in Podiatric Medicine for his academic contributions to medicine. David was Dean of the Faculty of Podiatric Surgery (2012-14) for the Royal College of Podiatry and has worked as an educational advisor to the Institute of Podiatry and, until 2024, was an affiliate with the University of Huddersfield, Human & Health Sciences.

Tim E Kilmartin

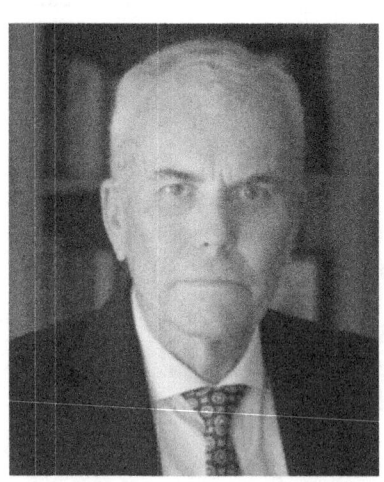

Tim has been a National Health Service Consultant Podiatric Surgeon since 1994. In that time, he has performed over 18,000 foot operations. He now works exclusively in private practice in Northern Ireland. Tim has published over ninety articles in national and international peer-reviewed journals on foot surgery and foot biomechanics. The cause and treatment of bunion problems remain a particular interest. Tim qualified in Birmingham in 1985 but went on to train in podiatric surgery in Northampton, Luton, Chicago and Seattle.

Tim completed a PhD on bunions in children at Nottingham University Medical School, Department of Orthopaedics, in 1994. He was the first Dean of the Faculty of Podiatric Surgery of the Royal College of Podiatrists, London. He is an adviser to the UK National Institute of Clinical

Excellence on foot joint replacements. He is also on the Editorial Board of the Journal of Foot and Ankle Research, The Foot, Journal of American Podiatric Medical Association and The Podiatrist. In 2023, Tim received the Diamond Award from the Royal College of Podiatry—the College's highest honour, awarded to individuals who have demonstrated substantial, outstanding, and exemplary contributions to the profession of podiatry over a sustained number of years.

Index

Books by the same authors at Amazon

Guide to Orthopaedic Conditions

Shoulder Pain—Rotator Cuff Repair. (2024)
Foot Health Myths, Facts & Fables. (2021)
Bunion. Hallux Valgus. Behind The Scenes. (2019)
Morton's Neuroma. Podiatrist Turned Patient. (2017)

Podiatry Career Books

Voices from Podiatric Medicine. (2023)
A Career in Podiatric Medicine. (2023)

Academic Books

The Foot. A Learning Companion. Workbook. (2024)
An Introduction to the Foot & Its Common Problems in the
Adult. (2023)
PowerPoint is More than A Slide Program. (2020)
Projecting Your Image. Conferences to Village Halls.
(2020)

Books also written with Tim E Kilmartin:-

Voices From Podiatric Medicine. Tollafield DR. (2023)
Assessment of the Lower Limb. Eds. Merriman &
Tollafield. Churchill-Livingstone. (1995)
Clinical Skills in Treating the Foot. Eds.Tollafield &
Merriman. Churchill-Livingstone. (1997)

The Complete Patient Guide To Bunion Problems.

Made in the USA
Las Vegas, NV
08 February 2025